KERATITIS

Edited by **Muthiah Srinivasan**

Keratitis
Edited by Muthiah Srinivasan

Published by InTech
Janeza Trdine 9, 51000 Rijeka, Croatia

Publishing Process Manager Jana Sertic

Technical Editor Teodora Smiljanic

Cover Designer InTech Design Team

Additional hard copies can be obtained from orders@intechopen.com

Keratitis, Edited by Muthiah Srinivasan
p. cm.
ISBN 978-953-51-0568-8

For EU product safety concerns:
IN TECH d.o.o., Prolaz Marije Krucifikse Kozulić 3, 51000 Rijeka, Croatia,
info@intechopen.com or visit our website at intechopen.com.

Meet the editor

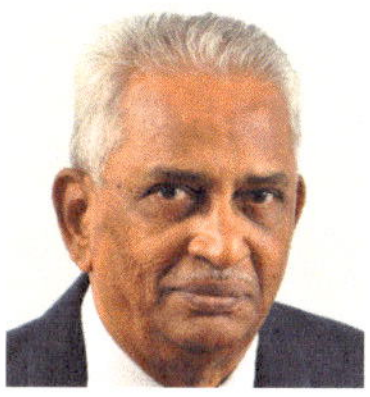

Dr. Muthiah Srinivasan, born on 9th May 1947 in India, completed medical school in 1972, Joined Aravind Eye Hospital and Post Graduate Institute of Ophthalmology, Madurai in 1981. He is currently serving as the Director – Emeritus and Prof. of ophthalmology in the same institute. He is expert in infectious diseases of cornea: prevention and managing corneal ulcer; corneal transplantation; eye banking; stem cell and refractive surgery. Dr. Srinivasan is serving as Medical Director of Rotary Aravind international Eye Bank, Madurai and Immediate Past President of Eye Bank Association of India. As a Postgraduate Teacher for the past 29 years, he has been invited to various conferences and Universities in India and abroad, received several awards including 2012 APAO, conducted several research studies, both clinical and epidemiological, including WHO sponsored studies in SEAR. The outcome of these studies provide evidence based management of the corneal diseases in developing world. He has published 136 papers in peer reviewed journals.

Contents

Preface

Readers may have access to several textbooks and peer reviewed journals about Keratitis, both in print and on-line versions. Recently due to advanced information technology made available even in developing nations; online publications have been viewed by several health professionals and public as a reliable source of information about health. This kind of publications works cheaper and could be shared by many users. Traditionally the title Keratitis covers non-infective and infective forms but the later one had been described elaborately in most of the languages. The contributing authors of this book have shifted their focus towards recent advances about Keratitis with their vast experience and expertise. Over the past few decades we have witnessed major expansion in the field of Keratitis and these chapters in this book will certainly improve the skill and knowledge of the readers involving patient management, clinical and basic research.

Keeping up with the broad advance in technology and treatment strategy is challenging but is essential if we are to utilize this knowledge effectively for patient care. As you open this book I hope you as a reader will appreciate the efforts of dedicated authors, reviewer and publisher to further enhancing the health science for better outcome.

Dr. Muthiah Srinivasan
Chief Medical Officer,
Aravind Eye Hospital and Postgraduate Institute of Ophthalmology,
India

1

An Overview of Fungal Keratitis and Case Report on Trichophyton Keratitis

Ivana Mravičić[1], Iva Dekaris[1], Nikica Gabrić[1], Ivana Romac[1], Vlade Glavota[1] and Emilija Mlinarić- Missoni[2]
[1]*University Depertment of Ophthalmology, Eye hospital „Svjetlost", Zagreb,*
[2]*Croatian National Institute of Public Health, Zagreb,*
Croatia

1. Introduction

1.1 Keratitis

Keratitis represents corneal inflammation from various causes and clinical manifestations. (Table 1.) It might affect populations of all ages, both males and females with variable incidence. The cornea has a few different defensive mechanisms because it is constantly exposed to external pathogens and enviromental influences:

- reflexive eye closing
- flushing effect of tearing
- epithelium diffusion barrier
- very quick regeneration ability

Due to impaired defensive mechanisms caused by injuries or little epithelial defects , different types of pathogens or environmental influences might induce corneal inflammation (keratitis). The form of corneal inflammation called superficial keratitis involves just the corneal surface (epithelium). If the inflammation involves corneal stroma it is called stromal or interstitial keratitis. Keratitis might be mild, moderate or severe and may involve other parts of the eye. It might be acute or chronic, infectious or noninfectious. All conditions that lead to epithelial break are possible risk factors to induce keratitis. Microorganisms cannot invade an intact, healthy cornea and infection rarely occurs in the normal eye because the human cornea is naturally resistant to infection.

Keratitis	
Noninfectious	**Infectious**
Superficial punctate keratitis	Bacterial keratitis
Exposure keratitis	Viral keratitis
Neuroparalytic keratitis	Fungal keratitis
	Protozoal keratitis

Table 1. Types of keratitis

1.1.1 Noninfectious keratitis

Noninfectious keratitis represents corneal inflammation with no known infectious cause. There is a wide spectrum of eye disorders that might be the very reason for this frequent corneal manifestation causing defects of corneal epithelium. This includes:

- tear film disturbances
- eyelid anomalies and inflammations
- physical or chemical trauma
- allergies
- problems with contact lens wearing
- facial neuropathy

Persisting epithelial defects are typically accompanied by this form of keratitis. Pain, tearing, redness, photophobia and decreased visual acuity are the most common clinical symptoms. Alongside symptomatic therapy, treatment also depends on the specific cause and it is aimed at promoting corneal healing.

1.1.2 Infectious keratitis

Infectious keratitis (microbial keratitis) as the most frequent cause of keratitis is a sight threatening process characterized by defects of corneal epithelium with inflammation of underlying corneal stroma. Bacteria, viruses, fungi and parasitic organisms are all possible causes of this medical emergency condition. The most common predisposing risk factors to develop infectious keratitis include overnight or extended contact lens wear, inadequate disinfection of contact lenses (contamination of the contact lens storage case or contact lens solution), trauma, previous ocular and eyelid surgery, especially corneal surgery (refractive surgery and keratoplasty), chronic ocular surface disease (tear film defficiencies , corneal exposure due to abnormalities of eyelid anatomy and function, systemic diseases (diabetes mellitus, immunocompromised status), extended use of topical corticosteroids. In about 10%of patients with infectious keratitis none of these risk factors was recognized. Clinical presentation varies and depends on the type of causative agent. Patients usually present with redness, tearing, rapid onset of pain and blurred vision. Varied physical findings can be revealed using slit lamp biomicroscopy and external examination will reveal : eyelid edema, conjunctival hyperemia , corneal ulceration, corneal infiltrates, stromal inflammation of the cornea, anterior chamber reaction with or without hypopion, Descemet folds, endothelial inflammatory plaques, posterior synechiae.

Infectious keratitis as a serious and possible eye threatening medical emergency requires prompt and adequate treatment. Treatment options include local and systemic antibacterial, antifungal and antiviral medications that depend on the underlying cause and severity of disease.

1.2 Fungal keratitis

Fungal keratitis or keratomycosis refers to an infective process of the cornea caused by any fungal species capable of invading the ocular surface. It is a result of fungal colonization or epithelial infiltration and/or invasion of the corneal stroma. It is most typically a slow, relentless disease that must be differentiated from other types of corneal conditions with similar presentation; especially its bacterial counterpart.

Fungal keratitis is a very serious, potentially sight-threatening corneal infection which most commonly develops in patients after trauma or those with a compromised corneal surface.

It is relatively rare. However, with the increasing and extensive use of antibiotics and corticosteroids there has been an increase in the incidence of fungal keratitis over the past 20 years. Worldwide, the reported incidence of fungal keratitis is 17% to 36%. Despite advances in diagnosis and medical treatment of keratomycosis, 15% to 27% of patients require surgical intervention such as keratoplasty, enucleation, or evisceration because of either failed medical treatment or advanced disease at presentation.

1.2.1 Etiology

Fungi are eukaryotic organisms that have rigid walls and multiple chromosomes containing both DNA and RNA.

They are either saprophytic, free organisms living out of decaying organic matter or pathological, those that need a living host for perpetuation. At least 35 genera of fungi have been reported and are associated with corneal infection, the more common among which are *Candida, Fusarium, Cephalosporium* and *Aspergillus.*

Keratomycosis can be caused by moulds (filamentous multicellular fungi that produce tubular projections known as hyphae): hyalohyphomycete (from any of the 30 genera with over 55 species) and pheohyphomycete (from 19 genera and over 30 species), or yeasts (unicellular fungi that reproduce by budding and may occasionally form hyphae or pseudo-hyphae) (from 7 genera, over 18 species).(Table 2).

Moulds		**Yeasts**
Hyalohyphomycetes	Pheohyphomycetes	
Fusarium spp.	*Alternaria* spp.	*Candida* spp.
Aspergillus spp.	*Curvularia* spp.	*Cryptococcus* spp.
Acremonium spp.	*Bipolaris* spp.	*Geotrichum* spp.
Paecilomyces spp.	*Cladosporium* spp.	*Malassezia* spp.
Penicillium spp.	*Lecytophora* spp	*Rhodotorula* spp.
Pseudallescheria boydii	*Phialophora* spp.	*Torulopsis* spp.
Verticillium spp.	*Phoma* spp.	*Trichosporon* spp.
Rhizopus spp.	*Aureobasidium* spp.	*Cryptococcus* spp.

Table 2. Most common agents of keratomycosis

The most common type of keratomycosis is **keratohyalohyphomycosis** caused by moulds of the *Fusarium* and *Aspergillus genera.* Some studies into the etiology of keratohyalohyphomycosis in the USA proved that species of the *Fusarium genus (F. solani* and *F. oxysporum,* in particular) were the causative agents in 64% of the cases. Species of *Aspergillus genus* (e.g. *A. fumigatus, A. flavus, A. niger*) rank second most frequent agents of keratomycosis. Other less common agents of keratohyalohyphomycosis belong to the following genera: *Acremonium, Cylindrocarpon, Paecilomyces, Penicillium, Pseudallescheria and Scopulariopsis. Zygomycete* moulds (genera *Absidia, Apophysomyces, Rhizopus*) are also documented agents of keratomycosis.

Keratopheohyphomycosis is a less common fungal infection of the cornea, more prevalent in tropical and subtropical regions, mostly caused by species of the genera *Curvularia, Alternaria, Bipolaris, Drechslera, Exserohilum* and *Phialophora.*

Moulds are responsible for most cases of fungal keratitis in tropical climates.

Yeasts rarely cause keramycosis, mostly species of the *Candida genus.* Risk factors for contracting **keratocandidosis** is a chronic disease of the cornea. Yeasts are responsible for most cases of fungal keratitis in temperate climates.

Causative agents of keratomycosis documented over the last five years by the Ministry of Health and Social Welfare Referal Center for mycological diagnostics or systemic and disseminated infections at the Croatian National Institute of Public Health, Zagreb, are species from the *Fusarium, Verticilium* and *Acremonium* genera. Extremely rare causative agents are primary pathogenic species of dermatophytic moulds eg. *Trichophyton spp.*

1.2.2 Pathogenesis

Fungal keratitis is more common in males than in females. Risk factors are previous history of ocular trauma (especially if organic matter is involved), agricultural occupations, age, pre-existing ocular disease, exposure keratopathy, chronic keratitis, hydrophillic contact lenses, chronic use of steroids, diabetes, systemic immunosuppressive disease.

Corneal trauma is the most frequent and major risk factor for fungal keratitis. There should be a high level of suspicion if a patient presents with a history of corneal trauma, particularly with plant or soil matter.Previous corneal trauma was documented in 26-100% of keratomycosis patients.

Fungal keratitis frequently occurs in farmers and outdoor workers after ocular injuries (sometimes trivial) involving some type of vegetable matter. It would appear that the fungus is inoculated into the cornea by the injuring material rather than by subsequent contamination of the epithelial defect by environmental organisms in most of the cases reported.

The trauma that accompanies contact lens wear is miniscule. Contact lenses are not a common risk factor of fungal keratitis. Candida is the principal cause of keratitis associated with therapeutic contact lense wear and filamentous fungi are the ones associated with refractive contact lens wear.

Environmental conditions including temperature, annual rainfall, windy seasons and the harvest period have a significant role in increasing the incidence. The incidence of fungal infections is higher in tropical and semitropical areas and is much more frequent in developing countries. In some hot and humid regions it accounts for 50% of cases.

Fungal keratitis is an important ophthalmic problem in all parts of the world, because it leads to corneal blindness and sometimes to loss of the eye.

Normal conjunctival microbiota usually does not consist of fungi. In some specific life or work circumstances, however, individuals are exposed to corneal trauma and thus become more prone to develop mycotic infection.

Corneal epithelium is firmly built and resistant to prospective invasion of microorganisms. The infection probably starts when the epithelial integrity is broken either due to trauma or ocular surface disease and fungi gain access into the tissue, proliferate and elicit a severe inflammatory response that can cause stromal necrosis and melting. Proteases, collagenases, and phospholipases, extracellular enzymes of moulds and yeasts facilitate their penetration into corneal stroma. These enzymes, fungal antigens and toxins liberated into the cornea can result with necrosis and damage of its architecture thus compromising the eye integrity and function. Once in the anterior chamber, the infection is very difficult to eradicate and aggressive surgery is usually required. Wearing safety glasses while gardening will diminish the risk of ocular trauma, also general hygiene, proper contact lens care and avoidance of nonessential steroid use should diminish the probability of mycotic infection.

Fungal keratitis was first described by Theodor Leber in 1879 in a farmer who had his cornea injured by wheat blades. The causative agent was *Aspergillus glaucus species*. Since then and until the middle of the last century, individual cases of keratomycosis caused by species of the *Aspergillus genus*, occurring through an injury of the cornea, were documented, mostly in the tropical regions. Whilst this entity is not a common cause of corneal infection, it certainly represents one of the major causes of infectious keratitis in tropical areas of the world.

The incidence of fungal keratitis has increased over the past 30 years as a result of the frequent use of ocular corticosteroids; a rise in the number of patients who are immuno-compromised, and the availability of laboratory diagnostic techniques that aid in its diagnosis.

Fungal keratitis, if not diagnosed and treated with celerity, can be rapidly destructive to the integrity of the eye, resulting in devastating ocular damage. Unfortunately,delayed diagnosis is common, primarily because of the lack of suspicion and even if the diagnosis is made accurately,management remains a challenge. Poor corneal penetration and limited commercial availability of antifungal drugs further exacerbate the management problem.

1.2.3 Clinical manifestations

Symptoms of fungal keratitis are similar to any corneal infection and include unilateral red eye, pain, foreign body sensation , photophobia, tearing, decreased vision and discharge. Pain and photophobia are initially mild, but become severe relative to the clinical signs.

The clinical appearance of fungal keratitis varies greatly depending on the duration and severity of infection.

Patients often have a history of trauma, chronic ocular surface disease or corticosteroid eye drop usage.

Signs vary with the infectious agent. In early disease there tends to be less redness and lid swelling than with bacterial infection. The corneal surface typically appears grey with a dry rough texture.

Non specific signs of fungal keratitis include conjunctival injection; epithelial defect; suppuration;stromal infiltration; anterior chamber reaction; hypopyon; aqueous flare and corneal neovascularization.

Specific signs of fungal keratitis include infiltrates with feathery margins, rough texture, raised borders, brown pigmentation, associated endothelial plaque, and satellite lesions; deep stromal infiltrates with an intact epithelium; dull grey appearance of the cornea with possible heaping of epithelium.

Sclerotic scatter can be used to highlight the density and scalloped borders of the fungal lesion. Many fungal ulcers demonstrate no striking morphological pattern, and often it is not possible to differentiate clinically between fungal keratitis and bacterial keratitis.

Filamentous keratitis is characterized by a grey-yellow stromal infiltrate with indistinct margins , a progressive infiltration, often surrounded by satellite lesions and hypopyon. Filamentous fungi classically grow in a feathery branching pattern, but may be very rapidly progressive and indistinguishable from bacterial keratitis. (Figure 1.)

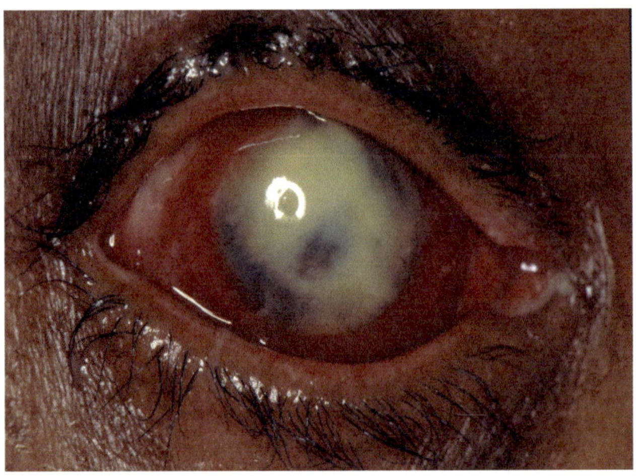

Fig. 1. Fungal corneal ulcer

Candida keratitis is characterized by a yellow-white infiltrate associated with dense suppuration. *Candida* species produces a small ulcer with expanding infiltrate in a collar-stud configuration, often superimposed on a debilitating corneal condition. There may be an endothelial plaque under the lesion and satellite lesions at the edges. Suppurative keratitis, fibrinoid uveitis, hypopyon and elevated IOP may occur.

Several features of fungal keratitis are characteristic if not pathognomonic and may permit an immediate or early diagnosis. These features are:

1. The surface of the lesion is usually gray or dirty white with a dry rough texture.
2. Areas of the lesion may be raised above the plane of the uninvolved cornea.
3. The margins of the ulcer tend to be irregular.
4. There may be satellite lesions.
5. There may be a complete or partial white immune ring" around the lesion. This is said to be formed by the fungal antigen and host antibody response.

1.2.4 Diagnostics

After establishing the patient's general condition the examiner should look for evidence of ocular surface disease. Determine the amount and type of secretions and lid swelling. The upper eyelid should be everted to exclude a retained foreign body. The examiner should measure the size and depth of the lesion as well as the presence of satellite lesions. Also the intraocular pressure should be ascertained. Anterior chamber reaction and evidence of hypopyon should be recorded. Vitreous reaction if present may suggest intraocular spread of the disease.

Under the slit lamp, early in the evolution, the lesion might look like an unhealed corneal abrasion with scanty infiltrates and no secretions. With time the ulcer develops thicker infiltrates and fuzzy margins. The presence of satellite lesions strongly suggests a fungal infection. Redness and periocular edema are also common. This combined with a history of trauma, especially with vegetable matter, ocular surface disease or chronic use of topical steroids should alert about the possibility of a mycotic etiology.

We should ask the patient about ocular or systemic disease: keratocandidosis is commonest in debilitated patients or those with preexisting corneal disease. Ocular trauma is associated with filamentous fungi, e.g. *Aspergillus* or *Fusarium spp.*

A diagnosis of fungal keratitis is based on a matrix of the following:

1. Case history
2. Clinical signs
3. Confirmation from cytology and/or culture results.

The most important step in the initial managment of suspected fungal keratitis is to obtain corneal material for direct smears and inoculation of media. It is important to scrape multiple sites in the ulcer crater, particularly at the margins, to enhance recovery of the organisms. Corneal scrapings are taken from deep into the lesion with a surgical blade or sterile spatula. To perform a corneal biopsy a dermatological 2 mm punch can be used.

Laboratory diagnostics should be performed before starting antifungal therapy. Filamentous fungi tend to proliferate anterior to Descement membrane and a deep stromal biopsy may be required (similar in technique to performing a trabeculectomy-the excised deep tissue is sent for culture). Sometimes the diagnosis can only be confirmed following anterior chamber tap or excisional keratoplasty.

Direct microscopy of corneal smears can be performed with special methods such as KOH, calcofluor white, Gram or/and Giemsa staining.. Gram stain may identify the yeast forms of Candida, and Giemsa stain is more likely to detect filamentous fungus.(Fig. 2)

Cultivation of causative agents can be done on Sabouraud´s dextrose agar, although most fungi will also grow on blood agar or in enrichment media at 27 deg celcius or at room temperature within 3 days. PCR with pan fungal primers are used as an adjunct to culture.

Antifungal susceptibility testing can be performed in reference laboratories but the relevance of these results to clinical effectiveness is uncertain.

Histology involving periodic acid-Schiff(PAS) stain and Grocott silver stain of corneal tissue are the most sensitive.

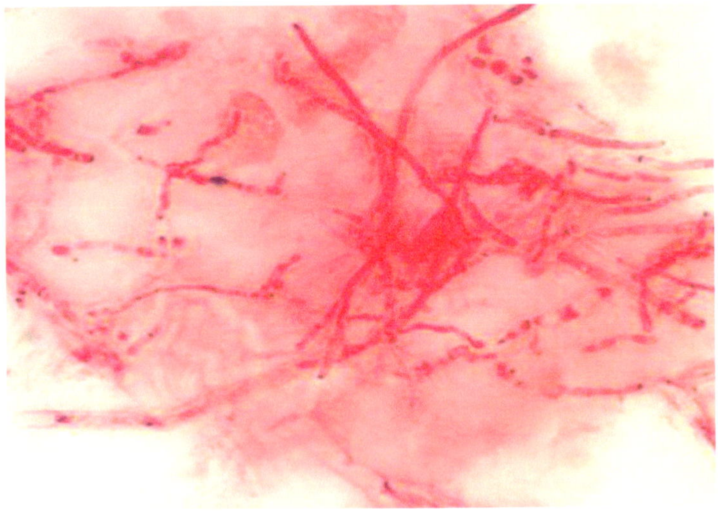

Fig. 2. Gram stain of corneal smear revealing hyphae

The drawback is that not all laboratories can handle those, so, again we might need to rely on the patient's evolution and the physician's clinical acumen. If all laboratory results are negative we should consider a corneal biopsy.

If available, in vivo confocal microscopy may be diagnostic.

1.2.5 Differential diagnosis

Fungal keratitis should be considered in the differential diagnosis of herpetic, acanthamoeba and atypical bacterial keratitis e.g. *Nocardia, Mycobacterium, Propionibacterium*; that does not respond to conventional treatment or has an unusual history or suspicious appearance.

1.2.6 Treatment

Antifungal therapy should be limited to cases with positive fungal smears or cultures. In general, management consists of medical therapy with the use of topical and or systemic anti-fungal medications alone or in combination with surgical treatment.

Antifungal agents are classified into the following groups:

- **Polyenes** include natamycin, nystatin, and amphotericin B. Polyenes disrupt the cell by binding to fungal cell wall ergosterol and are effective against both filamentous and yeast forms. Amphotericin B is the drug of choice to treat patients with fungal keratitis caused by yeasts. Although polyenes penetrate ocular tissue poorly, amphotericin B is the drug of choice for treatment of fungal keratitis caused by Candida. In addition, it has efficacy against many filamentous fungi. Administration is every 30 minutes for the first 24 hours, every hour for the second 24 hours, and then is slowly tapered according to the clinical response. Natamycin has a broad-spectrum of activity against filamentous organisms. The penetration of topically applied amphotericin B is found to be less than that of topically applied natamycin through the intact corneal epithelium. Natamycin is the only commercially available topical ophthalmic antifungal preparation. It is effective against filamentous fungi, particularly for infections caused by Fusarium. However, because of poor ocular penetration, it has primarily been useful in cases with superficial corneal infection.

- **Azoles** (imidazoles and triazoles) include ketoconazole, miconazole, fluconazole, itraconazole, econazole, and clotrimazole. Azoles inhibit ergosterol synthesis at low concentrations, and, at higher concentrations, they appear to cause direct damage to cell walls. Oral fluconazole and ketoconazole are absorbed systemically with good levels in the anterior chamber and the cornea; therefore, they should be considered in the management of deep fungal keratitis. Imidazoles and triazoles are synthetic chemical antifungal agents. High cornea levels of ketoconazole and fluconazole have been demonstrated in animal studies. Because of excellent penetration in ocular tissue, these medications, given systemically, are the preferred treatment of keratitis caused by filamentous fungi and yeast. The adult dose of ketoconazole is 200-400 mg/d, which can be increased to 800 mg/d. However, because of the secondary effects, increasing the dose should be done carefully. Gynecomastia, oligospermia and decreased libido have been reported in 5-15% of patients who have been taking 400 mg/d for a long period. The potential role of itraconazole in treatment of fungal keratitis is still unclear. However, it may be a helpful adjunctive agent in fungal keratitis. An oral antifungal (e.g. ketoconazole, fluconazole) should be considered for patients with deep stromal infection. Antifungal therapy usually is maintained for 12 weeks, and patients are monitored closely. Fluconazole has been shown to penetrate better into the cornea after systemic administration compared to other azoles and may be associated with fewer adverse effects.
- **Fluorinated pyrimidines**, such as flucytosine, are other antifungal agents. Flucytosine is converted into a thymidine analog that blocks fungal thymidine synthesis. It is usually administered in combination with an azole or amphotericin B; it is synergistic with these medications. Otherwise, if flucytosine is the only drug used in therapy for candidal infections, emergence of resistance rapidly develops. Therefore, flucytosine should never be used alone. Treatment should be instituted promptly with topical fortified antifungal drops, initially every hour during the day and every 2 hours over night. Subconjunctival injections may be used in patients with severe keratitis or keratoscleritis. They also can be used when poor patient compliance exists.

In vitro antifungal susceptibility testing is often performed to assess resistance patterns of the fungal isolate. However, in vitro susceptibility testing may not correspond with in vivo clinical response because of host factors, corneal penetration of the antifungal drug and difficulty in standardization of antifungal sensitivities. Therefore, they should be performed in a standardized method at a reference laboratory.

The promotion of fungal growth by corticosteroid treatment is well recognized; therefore, corticosteroid drops should not be used in the treatment of fungal keratitis until after 2 weeks of antifungal treatment and clear clinical evidence of infection control. Steroids should only be used when the active inflammation is believed to be causing significant damage to the structure of the cornea and/or vision. The steroid is always used in conjunction with the topical antifungal. Therapy may be modified. Decisions about alternate therapy must be based on the biomicroscopic signs and on the tolerance of the topical medications. Improvement in clinical signs may be difficult to detect during the initial days of antifungal therapy. However, some of the biomicroscopic signs that may be helpful to evaluate efficacy are as follows:

- Blunting of the perimeters of the infiltrate
- Reduction of the density of the suppuration
- Reduction in cellular infiltrate and edema in the surrounding stroma
- Reduction in anterior chamber inflammation
- Progressive reepithelization
- Loss of the feathery perimeter of the stromal inflammation

Successful antifungal therapy for fungal keratitis requires frequent drug administration for prolonged periods (ie, at least 12 wk). Some corneal manifestations of toxicity are as follows:

- Protracted epithelial ulceration
- Punctuate corneal epithelial erosion
- Diffuse stromal haze

Surgical therapy may be required not only for complications of acute infectious processes, but also if medical management fails.

Debridment

Debridement is the simplest form of surgical intervention. The organisms and necrotizing material is removed and the penetration of antifungal medications is enhanced by the removal of the epithelium, which is a barrier for the topical antifungals. Debridement is recommended only in cases when necrotic tissue unables healing of the corneal ulcer.

Biopsy

A biopsy is indicated for the direction of diagnostic and/or therapeutic treatment.

Conjuntival flaps

Conjunctival flaps have been advocated for nonhealing ulcers and are often effective, although fungal organisms have been found to persist under a conjunctival flap.

Penetrating keratoplasty (PK)

Penetrating keratoplasty should be performed sooner rather than later in cases not responding to aggressive antifungal therapy. If the infectious process progresses and the fungus reaches the limbus or sclera, it will be too late for keratoplasty to rid the eye of viable fungus, and the eye will be destroyed by the fungal infection.

Lamellar keratoplasty

Lamellar keratoplasty may be ineffective in treating fungal keratitis because of the inability to remove the infectious agent. If the area of infection can be completely encompassed by the penetrating graft, and if there has been an inadequate response to medical treatment, the corneal graft may be an effective cure.

Typically, diagnosis occurs late, as many practitioners frequently misdiagnose fungal keratitis as bacterial keratitis. Fungal keratitis is considered only after a presumed bacterial keratitis worsens during antibiotic therapy. Fungal keratitis is difficult to treat for various reasons. Few antifungal medications have good corneal penetration, and most are merely fungistatic hence requiring an intact immune system and a prolonged therapeutic course. Except for natamycin 5%, all antifungal medications must be adapted for ophthalmic use from systemic drugs. The result is considerable ophthalmic toxicity.

The three major goals for treating fungal keratitis are:

1. Eradicate the fungal infection
2. Prevent secondary bacterial infection
3. Control ocular pain

Analgesic therapy includes cycloplegics and nonsteroidal anti-inflammatory drugs. Atropine 1% ophthalmic solution or ointment should be applied topically, as frequently as is necessary, to maintain pupillary dilation. It not only blocks painful cilliary spasm but also minimizes the development of synechiae. Ocular pain may also be controlled by the systemic administration of non-steroidal anti-inflammatory drugs. Secondary glaucoma may require oral carbonic anhydrase inhibitors or hyperosmotic agents. Additional antibacterial therapy for individual cases should be guided by culture and sensitivity testing results. Because secondary bacterial invasion is likely, topical antibiotics should be included in the therapeutic regimen. Initial antibacterial therapy should be directed against both gram-positive and gram-negative organisms. Medical treatment can be effective, provided that suitable drugs are administered appropriately. Combinations of surgical and medical treatment usually reduce the duration of therapy, although surgical treatment can produce more scaring. Surgery is often chosen because of the shorter recovery time and potential better prognosis.

If the smear and cultures are negative at 48 to 72 hr in a patient with strong suspicion of having fungal infection, and the patient is not improving on the initial, broad- spectrum antibacterial therapy chosen, a corneal biopsy is required. If the corneal biopsy is still negative, the destructive corneal process is progressing, and hypopyon exists; anterior chamber paracentesis or excisional biopsy (keratoplasty) should be performed.

Adverse results range from mild to severe corneal scarring, corneal perforation, anterior segment disruption and glaucoma up to endophthalmitis resulting in evisceration. The aftermath of fungal keratitis can be dreadful. There is severe visual loss in 26% to 63% of patients. Fifteen to twenty percent may need evisceration. Penetrating keratoplasty is performed in 31 to 38%.

2. Case report

We present a 22 year-old female who developed a corneal ulcer after contact lens wearing. The patient was treated with topical antibiotics, the conjunctival swab was sterile but the patient developed corneal melting syndrome. She was continually treated with topical and systemic antibiotics for two weeks but then developed descemetocella with spontaneous corneal perforation and complicated cataract of the left eye as a complication of keratitis.

At that stage of the disease the patient was examined in our clinic for a second opinion (Figure 3). Immediately after she was admitted to our clinic, a conjunctival swab, a piece of corneal tissue and a sample from the anterior chamber were sent to the microbiology department for analysis. During the procedure, a lavage of the anterior chamber with cefuroxime and vancomycin was performed. Therapeutic urgent perforating keratoplasty (PK) was performed 48 hours after she was admitted into our clinic by placing the graft onto a healthy recipient part of the cornea together with extracapsular cataract extraction and the implantation of the intraocular lens in the posterior chamber (figure 4). Intraoperatively we found a melted cornea, descemetocella with central perforation, white-yellow snow balls in the anterior chamber with a thick pupilary membrane. The patient was treated with 400 mg i.v. ciprofloxacin and 50 mg diflucan, dexamethasone, atropine (subconjunctival application) and chlorhexidine, brolene, levofloxacin, polimyxin B, and dexamethasone/neomycin drops. Antibiotics were used because the results of culture and biopsy of corneal tissue and a sample from the anterior chamber were inconclusive. Use of antibiotics to prevent secondary bacterial infection in case of fungal keratitis is not generally advised unless the result of antibacterial swab is inconclusive. After the repeated swabs showed no bacterial ingrowth, systemic antibiotics were stopped.

Microbiological evaluation was performed following excisional biopsy of the intracameral portion of the lesion. The presence of *Trichophyton spp.* was confirmed. According to the infectologist's advice, 100 mg bid itraconazole was included in the systemic therapy. The corneal graft was clear for 17 days and then started to opacify and was rejected in the following 10 days. In spite of local and systemic therapy, microorganisms invaded the vitreous and caused endophthalmitis. Pars plana vitrectomy was performed in order to take fresh samples and decrease the quantity of microorganisms. In the postoperative period antifungal treatment was continued intensively. Despite the intensive therapy, the corneal graft gradually melted and the anterior chamber was again filled with inflammation masses. Anterior chamber washout with cefuroxim was done once again and samples were taken and sent to evaluation. *Trichophyton spp.* was confirmed but in decreased quantity. Due to progression of corneal melting, an amniotic membrane was transplanted to prevent perforation. In spite of systemic and local therapy, the patient developed endophthalmitis again and lost light sensation. Few months afterwards she developed phthysis. Evisceration with a drainage system was performed and a silicon prosthesis was implanted.

The patient had no macroscopic signs of mycotic infection in nails, foot or skin so the samples from this areas were not sent on microbiological evaluation. This patient worked in nursing home so she might had been in contact with patients who had dermatophytosis.

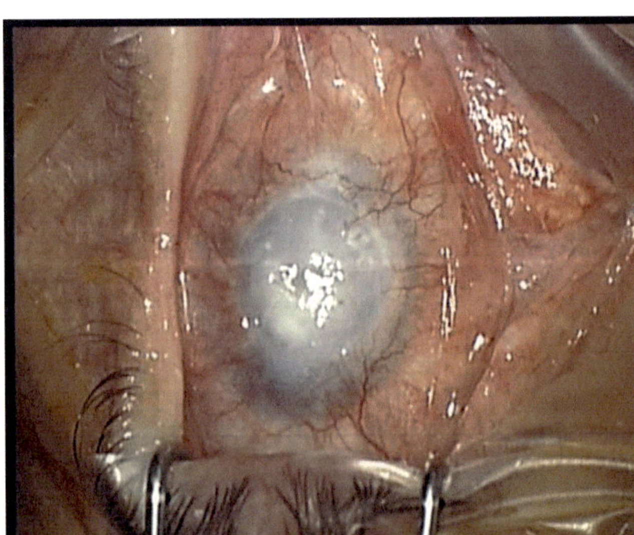

Fig. 3. Corneal ulcer developed after contact

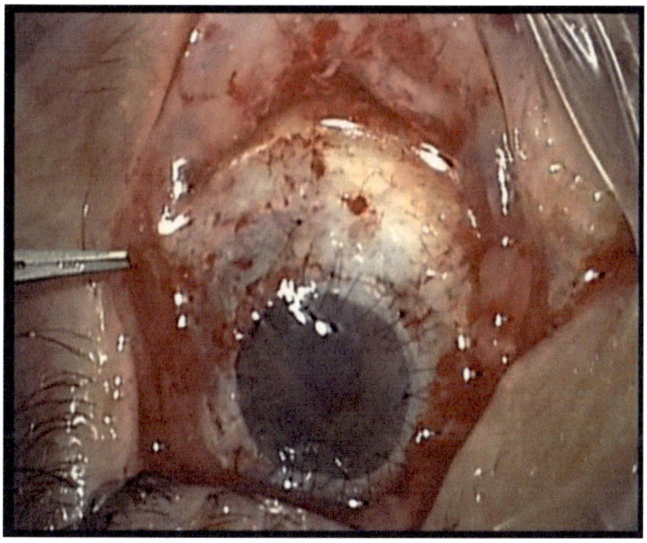

Fig. 4. Corneal graft after perforating keratoplasty lens wearing

3. Conclusion

Trychophyton spp. is a rare cause of fungal keratitis which can be associated with progressive keratolysis and corneal perforation. Severe disease of the anterior eye segment can extend to the posterior pole with endophthalmitis and consequentially can often end with the loss of vision or even the entire eye. Treatment can be medicamentous or surgical. There are several guidelines for the antifungal medicamentous treatment, but efficacy of currently available antifungal agents is limited and there is a relatively high medical treatment failure rate. Daily „debridment" with a spatula or blade can be performed due to removal of necrotic tissue which unables healing of the corneal ulcer, although it is not recommended if it is not necessary. Excimer laser **Phototherapeutic Keratectomy** (PTK) can be used for treating superficial infections. The most common surgical procedure is therapeutic penetrating keratoplasty. Keratoplasty is a method of choice when medical treatment fails or in the case of recurrent infection. It is wise to perform keratoplasty before infectious processes progress into the anterior chamber or before limbus or sclera are involved. The size of trephination should be planned to leave at least a 1 to 1.5 mm clear zone of clinically uninvolved cornea. Interrupted sutures should be used. Every affected intraocular structure (lens, iris, vitreous) should be excised and irrigation performed. If endophthalmitis is suspected antifungal agents should be injected intraoculary. After perforating keratoplasty topical antifungal agents shold be continued in combination with systemic antifungal therapy. Prompt diagnosis and treatment of fungal infection (in our case Trichophyton keratitis) is crucial for preservation of an eye for a good visual outcome.

4. References

Ajello, L; Hay, R.J.(1998). Medical Mycology. In: Topley & Wilson's Microbiology and Microbial infections.Arnold, London.

Dahl A.A. (2010). Keratitis, In: MedicineNet.com,Ac 22.8.2011., Available from:

De Hoog, GS et al.(2009). Atlas of Clinical Fungi. Centraalbureau voor Schimmelcultures: Utrecht.
http://emedicine.medscape.com/article/1194028-overview#showall
http://www.medicinenet.com/script/main/art.asp?articlekey=119219

Inderjeet Y.(2007). Review of fungal keratitis.

Jackson, T.L. Moorfields Manual of Ophthalmology, Mosby Elsevier.

Kanski, J.J.Clinical ophthalmology A systematic approach.

Lang, G.K. (2007). Ophthalmology (second edition), Georg Thieme Verlag, ISBN 3-13-126162-5, Stuttgart, Germany

Mlinarić-Missoni, E. (2009). Keratomikoza. In: Uzunović-Kemberović S. Medicinska mikrobiologija. Štamparija Fojnica d.o.o.: Fojnica.

Mravičić, I.; Dekaris, I.; Gabrić, N.; Romac, I.; Glavota, V.; Sviben, M.(2010) Trichophyton spp. fungal keratitis in 22 years old female contact lenses wearer. Coll Antropol; 34 (suppl 2): 271-4.

Murillo-Lopez F.H. Bacterial Keratitis, In: Medscape.com, 25.08.201., Available from:

Rapuano, C.J; Heng, W-J. Color Atlas&Synopsis of clinical ophthalmology Wills Eye Hospial „Cornea"

Richardson, MD; Johnson EM.(2006). Fungal infection. Blackwell Publishing: Oxford.

Shokohi, T.; Nowroozpoor-Dailami, K.; Moaddel-Haghighi T (2006). Fungal keratitis in patients with corneal ulcer in Sari, Northern Iran. Arch Iranian Med, 9(3):222-227.

Srinivasan, M. (2004). Fungal keratitis. Current Opinion in Ophthalmology, 15:321-327.

Thomas P.A., Geraldine P.(2007). Infectious keratitis. Current opinion in infectious diseases, 20(2) (Apr 2007), 129-41.

2

Bacterial Keratitis – Causes, Symptoms and Treatment

Hadassah Janumala, Praveen Kumar Sehgal and Asit Baran Mandal
Central Leather Research Institute
India

1. Introduction

The human eye is a complex organ of vital importance for everyday life. Eyes are the parts of our body that perceive light to see the world and to understand how objects relate to each other. We can distinguish far objects from close ones and determine their color and shape (Figure 1). The cornea is the dome-shaped window in the front of the eye. When looking at a person's eye, one can see the iris and pupil through the normally clear cornea. The cornea bends light rays as a result of its curved shape and accounts for approximately two-thirds of the eye's total optical power, with the lens of the eye contributing the remaining one-third. The cornea is as smooth and clear as glass but is strong and durable (Figure 2). It helps to shield the rest of the eye from germs, dust, and other harmful matter. The cornea shares this protective task with the eyelids, the eye socket, tears, and the sclera, or white part of the eye. A very thin tear film lies between the front of the cornea and our environment. The cornea copes very well with minor injuries or abrasions. If the highly sensitive cornea is scratched, healthy cells slide over quickly and patch the injury before infection occurs and vision is affected.

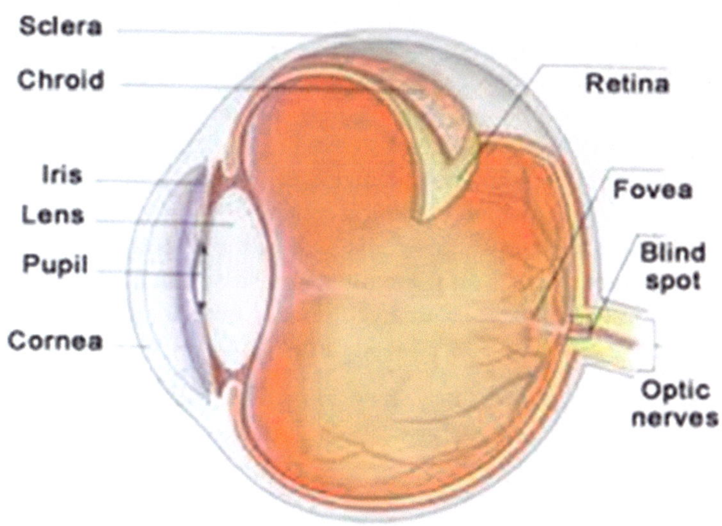

Fig. 1. Structure of the eye

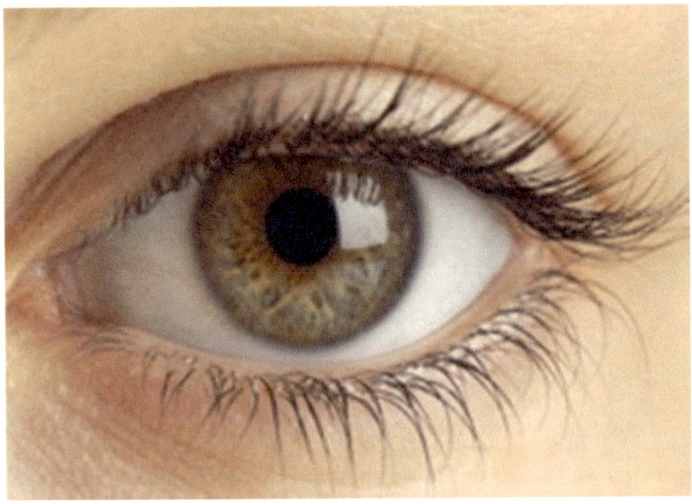

Fig. 2. Cornea is the clear part of the eye that covers the pupil

Bacterial keratitis is an infection and inflammation of the cornea that cause pain, reduced vision, light sensitivity and tearing or discharge from the eye that can, in severe cases cause loss of vision. Bacterial keratitis progresses rapidly and corneal destruction may be complete in 24 - 48 hours with some of the more virulent bacteria. The severity of the corneal infection usually depends on the underlying condition of the cornea and the pathogenicity of the infecting bacteria. It may involve the center of the cornea or the peripheral part of the cornea (that portion closest to the sclera) or both. Keratitis may affect one eye or both eyes. Keratitis may be mild, moderate, or severe and may be associated with inflammation of other parts of the eye (Figure 3). Keratitis can be classified by its location, severity, and cause. If keratitis involves the surface (epithelial) layer of the cornea, it is called superficial keratitis. Kerato-conjunctivitis is inflammation of the cornea and the conjunctiva. Kerato-uveitis is inflammation of the cornea and the uveal tract, which consists of the iris, ciliary body, and choroid. Keratitis may be acute or chronic. It may occur only once or twice in an eye or be recurrent. It may be limited in its effects on the eye or be progressive in its damage. Bacterial keratitis is a sight-threatening process. Many patients have a poor clinical outcome if aggressive and appropriate therapy is not promptly initiated. Some cases of keratitis results from unknown factors. Until recently, most cases of bacterial keratitis were associated with ocular trauma or ocular surface diseases. Various types of infections, dry eyes, injury, and a large variety of underlying medical diseases may all lead to keratitis.

Dry eye syndrome (DES; keratoconjunctivitis sicca) is a disorder of the tear film due to tear deficiency or excessive evaporation, which cause damage to the ocular surface. (Holly et al., 1977; Janumala H et al., 2009, 2010; Lemp et al., 1998; Tsubota et al, 1996) The signs of DES include foreign body sensation, ocular discomfort (scratchy, dry, sore, gritty, burning sensations) and problems with visual acuity. (Stern et al., 1998; Tsubota et al., 1992) Bacterial keratitis accounts for approximately 65% to 90% of all corneal infections. (Marios et al., 2007)

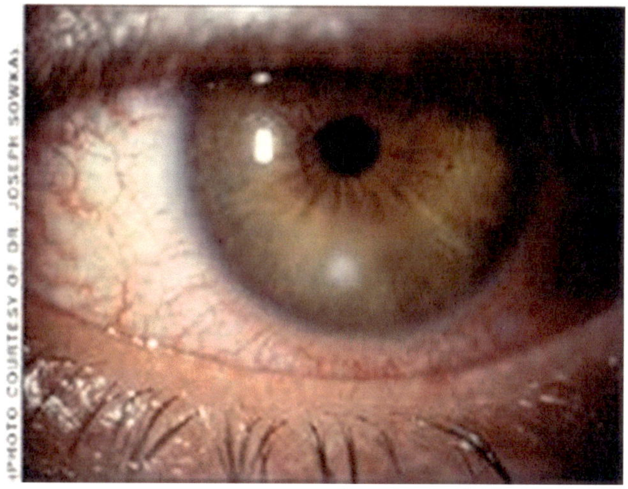

Fig. 3. Human eye with non-ulcerative Bacterial Keratitis

The spectrum of bacterial keratitis can also be influenced by geographic and climatic factors. Many differences in keratitis profile have been noted between populations living in rural or in city areas, in western, or in developing countries. Ulcerations of the cornea may occur, a condition known as ulcerative keratitis. Before the advent of antibiotics, syphilis was a frequent cause of keratitis. Corneal ulceration, stromal abscess formation, surrounding corneal edema, and anterior segment inflammation are characteristic of this disease. There are several types of keratitis, including superficial punctate keratitis, in which the cells on the surface of the cornea die; interstitial keratitis, a condition that can be either the direct result of infection, or more commonly secondary to an immunologic process; herpes simplex viral keratitis, caused by the sexually transmitted herpes virus; and traumatic keratitis, which results when a corneal injury leaves scar tissue. Early diagnosis and treatment is the key to minimizing any visual-threatening sequelae. In addition, close follow-up, attention to laboratory data, and changing antimicrobials if no clinical improvement is evident are important elements for successful outcome. The severity of the corneal infection usually depends on the underlying condition of the cornea and the pathogenicity of the infecting bacteria. Many patients have a poor clinical outcome if aggressive and appropriate therapy is not promptly initiated. (Acharya et al., 2009; Tang et al., 2009)

1.1 Epidemiology frequency

The most common predisposing factor for keratitis in southeast Brazil is trauma, especially corneal injury due to vegetation; observation clearly connected with following risk factors. The risk of agricultural predominance and vegetative corneal injury in fungal keratitis and associated ocular diseases in bacterial keratitis increase susceptibility to corneal infection. A hot, windy climate makes fungal keratitis more frequent in tropical zones, whereas bacterial keratitis is independent of seasonal variation and frequent in temperate zones. In tropical countries the incidence of bacterial keratitis is pathogens and show geographical variation in their prevalence. Thus, the spectrum of microbial keratitis varies with geographical location influenced by the local climate and occupational risk factors. In United States Approximately 25,000 Americans develop bacterial keratitis annually. International incidence of bacterial keratitis varies considerably, with less industrialized countries having a significantly lower number of contact lens users and, therefore, significantly fewer contact lens-related infections. Mortality/Morbidity in cases of severe inflammation, a deep ulcer and a stromal abscess may coalesce, resulting in thinning of the cornea and sloughing of the infected stroma.

2. Causes of bacterial keratitis

Keratitis can lead to vision loss from corneal scarring. Physical or chemical trauma is a frequent cause of keratitis. If the cornea is hit and damaged by a foreign body (a finger nail, an arm, a metal splinter or through contact lenses), can cause a scratch to the cornea. Scratches are usually harmless and not very deep, but they give bacteria and viruses the possibility of attacks, which gives the cornea inflammation and should therefore be detected and treated. There are various types of keratitis, but most commonly it occurs after an injury to the cornea, dryness, inflammation of the ocular surface or contact lens wear. A wide variety of conditions can lead to inflammation of the cornea. Among them are viral, bacterial, or fungal infections; exposure to ultraviolet light such as sunlight or sunlamps; exposure to other intense light sources such as welding arcs or snow or water reflections; irritation from excessive use of contact lenses; dry eyes caused by an eyelid disorder or insufficient tear formation; a foreign object in the eye; a vitamin A deficiency; or a reaction to eye drops, eye cosmetics, pollution, or airborne particles such as dust, pollen, mold, or yeast. The condition is also a side effect of certain medications. Bacterial keratitis remains one of the most important potential complications of contact lens use and refractive corneal surgery. "Organisms can infiltrate an intact cornea of a lens-wearer, and a biofilm can form on the contact lens. Interruption of an intact corneal epithelium and/or abnormal tear film permits entrance of microorganisms into the corneal stroma, where they may proliferate and cause ulceration or secondary effect or molecules and cause infection. The epithelium and stroma in the area of injury and infection swell and undergo necrosis. Acute inflammatory cells (mainly neutrophils) surround the beginning ulcer and cause necrosis of the stromal lamellae. The collagen of the corneal stroma is poorly tolerant of the bacterial and leukocytic enzymes, and undergoes degradation, necrosis and thinning. This leads to scarring of the cornea. As thinning advances, the cornea may perforate, thus introducing bacteria into the eye with ensuing endophthalmitis. Corneal infections rarely occur in the normal eye. They are a result of an alteration in the cornea's defense mechanisms that allow bacteria to invade when an epithelial defect is present. The organisms may come from the tear film or as a contaminant from foreign bodies, contact lenses or irrigating solutions. The severity of the disease depends on the strain of the organism, the size of the inoculums, the susceptibility of the host and immune response, the antecedent therapy and the duration of the infection. The process of corneal destruction can take place rapidly (within 24hrs with virulent organisms) so that rapid recognition and initiation of treatment is imperative to prevent visual loss.

Contact lens users are at an increased risk of corneal ulcers (Figure 4, Figure 5). The annual incidence of bacterial keratitis with daily-wear lenses is 3 cases per 10,000. Contact lens is the leading cause of corneal inflammation, and if we as a contact lens user experience the following symptoms should seek medical attention right away. The injury may become secondarily infected or remain noninfectious. Retained corneal foreign bodies are frequent sources of keratitis. (Dart et al., 1988; Liesegang et al 1997; Moriyama et al., 2008; Musch et al 1983; Poggio et al., 1989; Weissman et al., 2002)

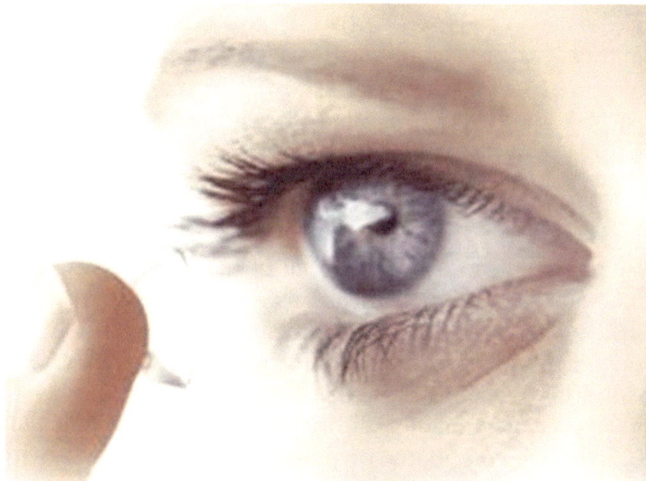

Fig. 4. Contact lens use

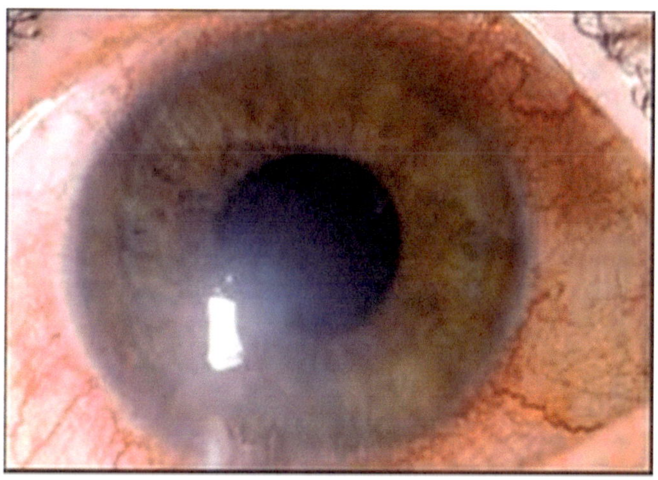

Fig. 5. Eye with keratitis infection due to contact lens use

2.1 Other causes for bacterial keratitis are

- Disturbances in the tear film may lead to changes in the corneal surface through drying of the corneal epithelium. This type of keratitis is usually superficial and most commonly is related to dry eyes and is known as keratitis sicca. If the eyes are extremely dry, the surface cells may die and form attached filaments on the corneal surface, a condition known as filamentary keratitis.
- Disorders that cause dry eyes; has no or limited germ fighting protection tears causing ulcers.
- Chemical solution splashes can injure the cornea and lead to corneal ulceration. Ultraviolet light from sunlight (snow blindness), a tanning light or a welder's arc, contact-lens over wear, and chemical agents, either in liquid form splashed into the eye or in gases in the form of fumes can all result in non-infectious superficial punctate keratitis,

- Inability to close the eyelids properly can also lead to cornea drying, including entropion with trichiasis and lagophthalmos a condition termed exposure keratitis.
- Allergies to airborne pollens or bacterial toxins in the tears may also cause a non-infectious type of keratitis. Autoimmune diseases create a similar appearance, often affecting the periphery of the cornea, termed marginal keratitis or limbic keratitis.
- Decreased immunologic defenses secondary to malnutrition, alcoholism, and diabetes (Moraxella).

Corneal ulcers are commonly caused by bacterial or fungal invasions following superficial corneal abrasions; among the common infectious agents are: staphyloccus, streptococcus, herpes (both simplex and zoster), adenovirus, rubeola, rubella, mumps, trachoma, infectious mononucleosis, and pneumococcus; also at fault may be Vitamin A deficiency or broad - spectrum antibiotic drug reactions. Corneal ulcers may also follow trauma, may be associated with other eye infections (e.g., conjunctivitis), may be related to other corneal disorders (e.g., degenerative conditions, or ptosis, which may cause a "dry eye"), or may arise from a variety of systemic disorders (especially those of autoimmune origin). In cases of severe inflammation, a deep ulcer and a stromal abscess may coalesce, resulting in thinning of the cornea and sloughing of the infected stroma. Once the corneal defenses are breached, specifically the epithelial glycocalyx, the cornea is prone to infection. Possible causes include direct corneal trauma, chronic eyelid disease, tear film abnormalities affecting the ocular surface and hypoxic trauma from contact lens wear. Pathogenic bacteria colonize the corneal stroma and immediately become antigenic, both directly and indirectly, by releasing enzymes and toxins. This sets up an antigen-antibody immune reaction that leads to an inflammatory reaction. The body releases polymorphonuclear leukocytes (PMNs) that aggregate at the area of infection, creating an infiltrate. The PMNs phagocytize and digest the bacteria. The collagen stroma is poorly tolerant of the bacterial and leukocytic enzymes and undergoes degradation, necrosis and thinning. This results in scarring of the cornea. With severe thinning the cornea may perforate, creating the possibility for endophthalmitis.

2.2 Gender

Males have a 30 to 40 per cent increased risk of developing keratitis compared to females. This gender difference has been reported previously for microbial keratitis. The reason for this association may be related to perceived health risks. Males have different attitudes and perceptions relating to health risks than do females, whereby they perceive risks as much smaller and much more acceptable. For example, males may be more inclined to underestimate the risk of developing corneal infiltrative events (CIE) when sleeping in contact lenses. (Efron et al., 2005a, 2005b, 2006; Morgan et al., 2005a, 2005b)

2.3 Smoking

Smoking was found to be associated with a 35 per cent greater risk of developing CIE's and this was increased to two-fold for severe keratitis. Others have reported similar findings. Smoking may be a risk factor for a number of reasons. It is generally considered that smoking is an unhygienic pursuit, which may be linked to a general lack of hygiene with respect to matters relating to contact lens wear and care. Toxins from smoke may either irritate the eyes directly or become absorbed into the contact lens and act as an irritant that compromises the health of the ocular surface and predisposes the eye to the development of corneal infiltrative events (CIE). Cigarette smoke is known to have an immuno-modulatory effect, which may indirectly predispose a cigarette smoker to develop a CIE.

2.4 Ocular and general health

Lens wearers have approximately twice the risk of developing a CIE in the absence of compromised ocular and general health. The protective effect of compromised ocular health in lowering the risk of contact lens associated CIEs may be explained by the precautionary attitude adopted by those with compromised ocular health in that such persons may cease lens wear, reduce wearing time or use self-prescribed topical ocular medications in an attempt to alleviate their condition. Such strategies might have the secondary effect of precluding the development of a CIE. An alternative explanation is that compromised ocular health may be associated with a general up- regulation of the innate defense status of the eye, so that there is an ever-present resistance to extraneous challenges to the ocular surface, which could result in a CIE. These principles can be extended to explain why compromised general health also serves to protect the eye from developing a CIE.

2.5 Season

The notion that adverse ocular conditions related to contact lens wear can be influenced by the time of year (seasonal effect) is well established; for example, Begley, Riggle and Tuel reported that the onset of contact lens-associated papillary conjunctivitis was seasonal, in that the incidence of this condition peaked during the allergy seasons in mid-western USA. We found a two to four times increased risk of developing CIEs in late winter (January to March in the northern hemisphere) compared with mid-summer (July in the northern hemisphere). We accessed the number of consultations for influenza-like illness to the United Kingdom National Health Service helpline by people aged 15 to 64 years in England during the same period as the Manchester Keratitis Study. This number peaked around October and November 2003, which is in disacordance with the peak incidence of CIEs in our study from January to March 2003. Interestingly, this observation is consistent with the finding of a lower incidence of CIEs in association with compromised general health. (Efron et al. 2006)

2.6 Risk of keratitis

In the Manchester Keratitis Study (Morgan et al 2005), logistic regression analyses were performed to investigate the association between a range of risk factors and the occurrence of CIEs. Daily wear of rigid lenses was found to be associated with a lower risk of developing CIEs compared with daily wear of hydrogel lenses. The risk of developing CIEs when sleeping in contact lenses is higher than in daily lens wear.

3. Symptoms of bacterial keratitis

The symptoms of keratitis usually include pain, tearing, and blurring of vision. The pain may be mild to severe, depending on the cause and extent of the inflammation. Sensitivity to light may also be present. To the observer, the eye may appear red, watery, and if the cornea has extensive keratitis, the normally clear cornea may look grey or have white to grey areas.

3.1 Physical

External and biomicroscopic examination of these patients reveal some or all of the following features: Ulceration of the epithelium; corneal infiltrate with no significant tissue loss; dense, suppurative stromal inflammation with indistinct edges; stromal tissue loss; and surrounding stromal edema. Increased anterior chamber reaction with or without hypopyon folds in the descemet membrane. Upper eyelid edema, Posterior synechiae surrounding corneal inflammation is either focal or diffuse, conjunctival hyperemia adherent mucopurulent exudate, endothelial inflammatory plaque.

A scratch on the cornea can cause

- Light annoyance.
- Blurred vision.
- Feeling "something in the eye".
- Pain

Cornea inflammation with bacteria cause

- Your eye turns red.
- Pain, impaired vision and sensitivity to light as a scratch.
- May be you see a gray-white speck in the eye (the pupil).

The patient will present with a unilateral, acutely painful, photophobic, eye. Visual acuity is usually reduced, and profuse tearing is common. There will be a focal stromal infiltrate with an overlying area of epithelial excavation. There is likely to be thick, ropy, mucopurulent discharge. The cornea will be very edematous. The conjunctival and episcleral vessels will be deeply engorged and inflamed, often greatly out of proportion to the size of the corneal defect. In severe cases, there will be a pronounced anterior chamber reaction, often with hypopyon. Intraocular pressure may be low due to secretory hypotony of the ciliary body, but most often will be elevated due to blockage of the trabecular meshwork by inflammatory cells. Often, the eyelids will also be edematous. Bacterial keratitis is a sight-threatening process. Bacterial keratitis makes the cornea cloudy. It may also cause abscesses to develop in the stroma, which is located beneath the outer layer of the cornea.

Interruption of an intact corneal epithelium and/or abnormal tear film permits entrance of microorganisms into the corneal stroma, where they may proliferate and cause ulceration. Virulence factors may initiate microbial invasion, or secondary effector molecules may assist the infective process. Many bacteria display several adhesions on fimbriated and non-fimbriated structures that may aid in their adherence to host corneal cells. During the initial stages, the epithelium and stroma in the area of injury and infection swell and undergo necrosis. Acute inflammatory cells (mainly neutrophils) surround the beginning ulcer and cause necrosis of the stromal lamellae. Diffusion of inflammatory products (including cytokines) posteriorly elicits an outpouring of inflammatory cells into the anterior chamber and may create a hypopyon. Different bacterial toxins and enzymes (including elastase and alkaline protease) may be produced during corneal infection, contributing to the destruction of corneal substance. The most common groups of bacteria responsible for bacterial keratitis are as follows: *Streptococcus, Pseudomonas, Enterobacteriaceae* (including *Klebsiella, Enterobacter, Serratia,* and *Proteus*), and *Staphylococcus* species.

3.2 Complications with keratitis

Irregular astigmatism: Another possible complication of these infections is uneven healing of the stroma, resulting in irregular astigmatism.

Corneal perforation: This is one of the most feared complications of bacterial keratitis that may result in secondary endophthalmitis and possible loss of the eye.

3.3 How is keratitis diagnosed?

Keratitis can be diagnosed by an ophthalmologist (a physician who specializes in diseases and surgery of the eye) by physical examination of the eye and history. The history consists of questions documenting a past medical and ocular history and the symptoms specific to the current visit. The eye examination will consist of checking the vision and careful inspection of the corneas using a slit lamp, which is a microscope with excellent illumination and magnification to view the ocular surface and the cornea in detail. In cases in which infection is suspected, a culture may be taken from the surface of the eye for specific identification of the bacteria, virus, fungus, or parasites causing keratitis. Slit lamp examination helps to diagnose the depth of the keratitis eye infection.

- Swab the eye or take samples from the eye to confirm the diagnosis of herpes simplex infection.
- Testing visual sharpness and clearness (visual acuity).
- Testing how well the pupil responds to light.
- Patients' history to know about any recent infection of the upper respiratory tract accompanied by cold sores.
- Blood tests may also be done in certain patients with suspected underlying disease.

3.4 What are the risk factors for keratitis?

- Major risk factors for the development of keratitis include any break or disruption of the surface layer (epithelium) of the cornea.
- The use of contact lenses increases the risk for the development of keratitis, especially in poor hygiene, improper solutions, or over wear of the lens.
- A decrease in the quality or quantity of tears predisposes the eye to the development of keratitis due to corneal drying.
- Disturbances of immune function through diseases such as AIDS or the use of medications such as corticosteroids or chemotherapy also increase the risk of developing keratitis.

3.5 Precautions and complications of corneal inflammation

If you have a job where you are exposed to metal pieces or similar things, you should wear goggles and visit a doctor when symptoms of a scratch on the cornea appear to prevent inflammation. Inflammation can spread deeper into the cornea and is difficult to treat. Therefore we should seek medical advice by herpes cornea inflammation every time. Bacteria can also produce a severe corneal inflammation, which in the worst case, permanent visual impairment. You must also not wear contact lenses before the eye has healed. If the scratch penetrates the cornea more deeply, however, the healing process will take longer, at times resulting in greater pain, blurred vision, tearing, redness, and extreme sensitivity to light. These symptoms require professional treatment. Deeper scratches can also cause corneal scarring, resulting in a haze on the cornea that can greatly impair vision. In this case, a corneal transplant may be needed.

4. Treatment of bacterial keratitis

Wound healing of the ocular surface is a special process due to its non-vascularity. It depends on surrounding corneal tissues for nourishment. Healing requires regeneration of the corneal and conjunctival epithelium, reduced scar formation, retention of transparency of cornea and mobility of the conjunctiva. Janumala H et al., 2009; Reim et al. 1997) The process of corneal wound healing consists of different phases, i.e. latent phase, cell migration, adhesion and

cell proliferation. Another fluoroquinolone, ofloxacin 0.3% (Ocuflox) is also an effective treatment for bacterial keratitis. Both fluoroquinolones are as effective at managing bacterial keratitis as fortified antibiotics, but with significantly fewer side effects. (Marios et al., 2007; Baker et al., 1996) Adjunctive use of cold compresses will also help to reduce inflammation. If there is evidence of secondary inflammatory glaucoma, Rx a topical beta-blocker BID. Have the patient return daily for follow-up visits. Once the infection is controlled, add a topical steroid Q2H to the regimen. Continue the daily follow-up and begin to taper all medications as you see improvement. (McLeod et al., 1995)

4.1 What is the treatment for keratitis?

Medical treatment is absolutely essential - even a delay of a few hours can affect the ultimate visual result. The causative factors must be determined through laboratory analysis of scrapings; medical treatment (i.e., medication) varies according to the cause. As with bacterial conjunctivitis, culturing the infection is the ideal way to determine the infecting organism but is often difficult or impractical. First and foremost, you must halt bacterial proliferation; do not delay treatment while waiting for the culture results. If you have the materials available, scrape the ulcer using a platinum spatula and plate the specimen into blood and chocolate agar culture media. A simpler but less effective method is to use a culturette. (McLeod et al 1996; Miedziak et al., 1999; Schaefer et al., 2001) Regardless, immediately begin therapy with a broad - spectrum antibiotic. A popular initial therapy is the fluoroquinolone ciprofloxacin 0.3% (Ciloxan) two drops every 15 minutes for six hours, followed by two drops every 30 minutes for 18 hours, and then tapered depending on patient response. Infectious keratitis generally requires antibacterial therapy to treat the infection. This treatment can involve prescription eye drops, pills, or even intravenous therapy. Any corneal or conjunctival foreign body should be removed. Wetting drops may be used if disturbance of the tears is suspected to be the cause of the keratitis. Steroid drops may often be prescribed to reduce inflammation and limit scarring. This must be done carefully and judiciously, since some infections can be worsened with their use. Treatment depends largely on the source of the problem. If a common adenoviral virus is causing the keratitis, the condition is likely to clear up on its own, usually in about two to three weeks. Available medications for this form of keratitis include palliative treatment. Contact-lens wearers are typically advised to discontinue contact-lens wear, whether or not the lenses are related to the cause of the keratitis.

4.2 Treatment of scratches on the cornea

- Foreign body should be removed if it sits in the eye.
- Antibiotics-drops to prevent inflammation.
- Possibly putting a small bandage over the eye in order to give it a little calm.

4.3 Keratitis antibiotic treatment

Staphylococcus aureus is a major cause of bacterial keratitis. (Alexandrakis et al., 2003; Liesegang et al. 1998) S. aureus ocular infections can cause severe inflammation, pain, corneal perforation, scarring, and loss of visual acuity. (Chusid et al., 1979) S. aureus has a long history of evolving to more resistant states, and this trend is expected to continue. (Hiramatsu et al., 1997; Peterson, 1999) Therefore, new antibiotics and new antibiotic formulations are needed to manage future cases of S. aureus-induced keratitis. Moxifloxacin and gatifloxacin are "fourth generation" fluoroquinolone antibiotics that target bacterial DNA gyrase (topoisomerase II) and topoisomerase IV. (Adams et al., 1992; Dalhoff et al., 1996; Kato et al., 1992; Shen, 1994) These fourth generation fluoroquinolones have in vitro activity similar to that of ciprofloxacin and ofloxacin (extended-spectrum fluoroquinolones) against gram-negative bacteria but enhanced activity against gram-positive bacteria, including S. aureus. (Biedenbach et al., 1996; Davis et al. 1994) A broadspectrum antibiotic may prevent secondary bacterial infection. Chronic dendritic keratitis may be effectively treated with vidarabine, long term topical therapy may be necessary. Keratitis due to exposure requires application of moisturizing ointment to the exposed cornea and protects it with eye patch. Severe corneal scarring may be treated by keratoplasty (cornea transplantation). Slit lamp photography can be useful to document the progression of the keratitis, A B-scan ultrasound can also be carried out in severe corneal ulcers with no view of the posterior segment. The fourth-generation ophthalmic fluoroquinolones include moxifloxacin and gatifloxacin and they are now being used for the treatment of bacterial conjunctivitis. Both antibiotics have better in vitro activity against gram-positive bacteria than ciprofloxacin or ofloxacin. Moxifloxacin penetrates better into ocular tissues than gatifloxacin and older fluoroquinolones; in vitro activity of moxifloxacin and gatifloxacin against gram-negative bacteria is similar to that of older fluoroquinolones. Polymicrobial keratitis has been reported in up to 12% of cases and can be difficult to treat. The use of multiple antibiotics simultaneously and with frequent dosing may result in added toxicity and damage to the ocular surface epithelium, thereby impairing recovery. Demonstration of broad-spectrum efficacy, excellent safety profiles in ocular infections, and a distinct mode of resistance acquisition. Moxifloxacin is a fourth-generation fluoroquinolone that exhibits a broad spectrum of bactericidal activity against both Gram-positive and Gram - negative bacterial pathogens, including staphylococci, *S. pneumoniae,* members of the family enterobacteriaceae, *P. aeruginosa, H. influenzae,* and *Moraxella* species. Moxifloxacin also has better mutant prevention characteristics than other fluoroquinolones. Moxifloxacin has also been shown to have superior activity compared with ciprofloxacin against quinolone resistant strains of *S. aureus.* Data also shows superior corneal and aqueous penetration of moxifloxacin (Solomon R, Donnenfeld E, et al.) Penetration of topically applied gatifloxacin 0.3%, moxifloxacin 0.5% and ciprofloxacin 0.3% into the aqueous humor.

4.4 Treatment with Succinylated Collagen Bandage lenses (SCBL)

Succinylated Collagen Bandage Lenses SCBL, are prepared with modified collagen (pH7.4) a natural biopolymer with biocompatibility with the human cornea, bioerodability, non-immunogenicity, high oxygen permeability, good water content, optimum thickness and superior physiological environment compared to hydrogel lenses. When used as a corneal adjunct in various conditions SCBL eliminates side effects such as irritation of the cornea, inflammation, watering, reduced visual acuity etc. SCBL shows promise to treat dry eyes, keratitis and epithelial trauma. (Janumala H et al.,2008, Janumala H et al., 2009)

4.5 Complications of keratitis?

Superficial keratitis involves the superficial layers of the cornea and commonly does not lead to scarring. More extensive keratitis involves deeper layers of the cornea, and a scar may develop upon healing. This will affect the vision if the central portion of the cornea is involved. With severe ulcerative keratitis, the cornea may perforate, which is an extremely serious situation. With proper diagnosis and appropriate treatment including follow-up care, keratitis can usually be managed without causing permanent visual disturbances. (Callegan et al., 1992; Davis et al. 1978) Vision often improves with treatment of the underlying infection. However, there may be some scarring of the cornea after treatment that may or may not affect vision in the long run. If the corneal scarring is in the center of the cornea, where it affects the line of site, a corneal transplant may ultimately be needed to improve the vision.

4.6 Can keratitis be prevented?

The risk of keratitis can be reduced through the use of safety precautions to avoid eye injury, and the prompt treatment of early ocular symptoms.

- Many forms of keratitis can be prevented by good hygiene.
- Protecting the cornea from injury is the first step, since keratitis also results from a corneal injury.
- If you have a cold sore or genital herpes, avoid touching the eyes.
- Have well balanced diet, including vitamin A rich foods such as carrots, squash, mangoes, sweet potatoes and spinach.

4.6.1 Prevention tips for contact lens users

- Contact lens users should always use sterile lens cleanser and disinfection solution.
- Do not over use contact lenses at night and make the eyes red or irritated.
- Never sleep with the contact lenses in the eyes.
- Always store the lenses in disinfecting solutions overnight.
- Regularly clean your contact lens case.
- Careful contact-lens care including proper cleaning of contact lens cases.

4.6.2 Keratitis home remedies

- A sterile, cotton-tipped applicator may be used to gently remove infected tissue and allow the eye to heal more rapidly.
- Can wear an eye patch to protect it from bright light and foreign particles.
- Minor infections are treated with antibacterial or antifungal eye drops.
- If keratitis is caused by dry eye, artificial tears for lubrication are effective.
- Vitamin supplementation such as vitamin A can be used in case deficiency is a suspected cause.

4.7 Clinical pearls

- If a patient presents with a corneal infiltrate but no overlying epithelial staining, the condition is not bacterial keratitis. If there is epithelial breakdown but only minor inflammation and anterior chamber reaction, then it is most likely not infectious bacterial keratitis.
- The inflammatory reaction is as damaging to the cornea as the infective organism. Once you've halted bacterial proliferation, be sure to prescribe a steroid to speed healing and reduce corneal scarring. For steroids to be beneficial, they must be used while the ulcer bed is still open, usually within the first 24 to 48 hours. If you wait until the ulcer re-epithelializes before adding a steroid, the beneficial effects will be lost.

5. Conclusion

- It is extremely important to treat keratitis before corneal tissue is destroyed and scar tissue is formed. Because the pain is so severe in keratitis, the patient usually welcomes medical attention. However, if the cornea loses its sensitivity (as in trauma, surgery, or damage to the trigeminal nerve), ulcers can develop without accompanying pain.
- The implications for personal hygiene are evident, especially with children. Hand washing *during* periods of illness and following toileting is of vital importance as a preventive measure.

6. Acknowledgements

I thank Dr. A. B. MANDAL, Director, CLRI-CSIR for his support to publish this book chapter. I am thankful to my husband Dr. Victor B. Kassey and my loving children Sharon Kassey, Angela Kassey and Daniel Kassey for their unconditional love, support and encouragement. Above all, I thank God for "*He has made everything beautiful in its time*" (Ecclesiastes 3:11).

7. References

Acharya, N.R., M. Srinivasan, J. Mascarenhas, *et al.* (2009) "The Steroid Controversy in Bacterial Keratitis." *Arch Ophthalmol.*, 127, 1231.

Adams, D. E., Shekhtman, E. M., Zechiedrich, E. L., Schmidt, M. B., & Cozzarelli, N. R. (1992), The role of topoisomerase IV in partitioning bacterial replicons and the structure of catenated intermediates in DNA replication. *Cell,* 71, 277-288.

Alexandrakis, G., Alfonso, E. C., & D. Miller. (2000), Shifting trends in bacterial keratitis in south Florida and emerging resistance to fluoroquino-lones, *Ophthalmology* 107, 1497-1502.

Baker, RS, Flowers, Jr. CW, Casey, R, *et al.* (1996) Efficacy of ofloxacin vs. cefazolin and tobramycin in the therapy for bacterial keratitis. *Arch. Ophthalmol,* 114, 632-633.

Biedenbach, D. J., & Jones, R. N. (1996), The comparative antimicrobial activity of levofloxacin tested against 350 clinical isolates of streptococci. *Diagn. Microbiol. Infect. Dis.* 25, 47-51.

Callegan, M. C., Hobden, J. A., Hill, J. M., Insler, M. S., & O'Callaghan R. J.(1992), Topical antibiotic therapy for the treatment of experi- mental Staphylococcus aureus keratitis, *Investig. Ophthalmol. Vis. Sci.* 33, 3017-3023.

Chusid, M. J., & S. D. Davis. (1979). Experimental bacterial keratitis in neutropenic guinea pigs: polymorphonuclear leukocytes in corneal host defense. *Infect. Immun.* 24, 948–952.

Dalhoff, A., Petersen, U., & Endermann, R. (1996), In vitro activity of BAY 12-8039, a new 8-methoxyquinolone. *Chemotherapy* 42, 410–425.

Dart, J.K. (1988), Predisposing factors in microbial keratitis: the significance of contact lens wear. *Br. J. Ophthalmol*, 72, 926–930.

Davis, R., & Bryson H. M. (1994), Levofloxacin. A review of its antibacterial activity, pharmacokinetics and therapeutic efficacy. *Drugs*, 47, 677–700.

Davis, S.D., Sarf, L.D., & Hyndiuk, R.A. (1978), Topical tobramycin therapy of experimental Pseudomonas keratitis: an evaluation of some factors which potentially enhance efficacy. *Archives of Ophthalmology*, 96, 123-125.

Efron, N, Morgan, P.B, Hill, E.A, Raynor, & MK, Tullo, A.B. (2005a), The size, location and clinical severity of corneal infiltrative events associated with contact lens wear. *Optom Vis. Sci.*, 82: 519–527.

Efron, N, Morgan, PB, Hill, EA, Raynor, & MK, Tullo. AB. (2005b), Incidence and morbidity of hospital-presenting corneal infiltrative events associated with contact lens wear, *Clin. Exp. Optom.*, 88, 232–239.

Efron, N., & Morgan, P.B. (2006) Impact of differences in diagnostic criteria when determining the incidence of contact lens associated keratitis, *Optom.Vis. Sci.*, 83, 152–159.

Hiramatsu, K., Aritaka, N., Hanaki, Kawasaki, H., S., Hosoda, Hori, Y., S., Fukuchi, Y., & Kobayashi, I. (1997), Dissemination in Japanese hospitals of strains of Staphylococcus aureus heterogeneously resistant to vancomycin. *Lancet* 350, 1670–1673.

Holly, F.J., & Lemp, M.A. (1977) Tear physiology and dry eyes, *Surv. Ophthalmol.*, 22, 69–87.

Janumala., H., Namita., B., Rao., U, & Sehgal., P. K. (2009), Evaluation of Succinylated Collagen Bandage Lenses in Corneal Healing by the Expression of Matrix Metalloproteinases (MMP-2 and MMP-9) in Tear Fluid, *Ophthalmic Res.*, 42, 64–72.

Janumala, H., Namita, B., Deepti, S., & Sehgal, P.K. (2010) Preparation and Clinical Evaluation of Succinylated Collagen Punctal Plugs in Dry Eye Syndrome - A Pilot Study, *Ophthalmic Res.* 43, 185–192.

Kato, J., Suzuki,H., & Ikeda, H. (1992), Purification and characterization of DNA topoisomerase IV in Escherichia coli, *J. Biol. Chem.* 267, 25676–25684.

Lemp, M.A, (1998) Epidemiology and classification of dry eye in lacrimal gland tear film and dry eye syndromes 2; in Sullivan D (Ed): Dartt DA, Meneray MA. New York, Plenum Press, pp 791–803.

Lemp, MA., (2000), Evaluation and differential diagnosis of keratoconjuctivitis sicca. *J. Rheumatol Suppl.*, 61, 11–14.

Liesegang, T.J. (1997), Contact lens-related microbial keratitis: Part I: Epidemiology, *Cornea*, 16, 125–131.

Liesegang, T.J. (1998), Bacterial and fungal keratitis, pp 159–219. In H. E. Kaufman (ed.), The cornea, 2nd ed. Butterworth-Heinemann, Boston, Mass.

Marios, C., Mark, D., Grant, R. S., Hien T. Vu, Hugh, R. Taylor, AC, (2007) Clinical Efficacy of Moxifloxacin in the Treatment of Bacterial Keratitis - A Randomized Clinical Trial, *Ophthalmology,* Vol. 114, Issue 9, pp 1622-1629.

McLeod, SD., LaBree, LD., & Tayyanipour, R., *et al.* (1995), The importance of initial management in the treatment of severe infectious corneal ulcers, *Ophthalmology,* 102, 1943–1948.

McLeod, S.D., Kolahdouz, I.A., & Rostamian, K., *et al.* (1996), The role of smears, cultures, and antibiotic sensitivity testing in the management of suspected infectious keratitis. *Ophthalmology,* 103, 23–8.

Miedziak, A.I., Miller, M.R., Rapuano, C.J., *et al.* (1999). Risk factors in microbial keratitis leading to penetrating keratoplasty, *Ophthalmology,* 106, 1166–1171.

Morgan, P.B, Efron, N, Brennan, NA, Hill, EA, Raynor, MK, Tullo, AB. (2005a) Risk Factors for the Development of Corneal Infiltrative Events Associated With Contact Lens Wear." *Invest Ophthalmol Vis. Sci.* 46, 3136-3143.

Morgan, PB, Efron, N, Hill, EA, Raynor, MK, Whiting, MA, Tullo, (2005b) AB. Incidence of keratitis of varying severity among contact lens wearers. *Br. J. Ophthalmol.,* 89, 430–436.

Moriyama, A. S., Hofling, A.L (2008) Contact lens-associated microbial keratitis, *Lima Arquivos Brasileiros de Oftalmologia* 71(6) , Suppl, pp 32-36.

Musch, DC, Sugar, A, Meyer, R.F. (1983) Demographic and predisposing factors in corneal ulceration. *Arch Ophthalmol,* 101, 1545–1548.

Peterson, D. L. (1999), Vancomycin-resistant Staphylococcus aureus. *Infect. Med.* 16, 235–238

Poggio, E.C., Glynn, R.J, & Schein, O.D. (1989), The Incidence of Ulcerative Keratitis Among Users of Daily-Wear and Extended-Wear Soft Contact Lenses, *N. Engl. J. Med.,* 321, 779-783.

Reim., M, Kottek., A, & Schrage, N. (1997), The cornea surface and wound healing, *Prog. Retinal Eye Res,* 16, 183–225.

Schaefer, F., Bruttin, O., & Zografos, L., *et al.* (2001) Bacterial keratitis: a prospective clinical and microbiological study. *Br. J. Ophthalmol.,* 85, 842–847.

Shen, L. L. (1994), Molecular mechanisms of DNA gyrase inhibition by quinolone antibacterials. *Adv. Pharmacol.* 29A, 285–304.

Stern, M.E., Beuerman, R.W., Fox, R.I., Gao, J., Mircheff, A.K., Plugfelder, S.C. (1998), The pathology of dry eye: the interaction between the ocular surface and lacrimal glands. *Cornea,* 17, 584–589.

Tang, A., Marquart, M.E., Fratkin, J.D., McCormick, C.C, Caballero, A.R, Gatlin, H.P, O'Callaghan, R.J. (2009). "Properties of PASP: a Pseudomonas protease capable of mediating corneal erosions". *Invest Ophthalmol Vis.* Sci. *50 (8): 3794–801.*

Tsubota, K., Yamada, M. (1992) Tear evaporation from the ocular surface, *Invest. Ophthalmol Vis. Sci.,* 33, 2942–2950.

Tsubota, K., Hata, S., Okusawa, Y., Egami, F., Oh- tsuki, T., Nakamori K. (1996) Quantitative video- graphic analysis of blinking in normal subjects and patients with dry eye, *Arch Ophthalmol,* 114, 715–720.

Weissman, B.A, Mondino, B.J. (2002), Risk factors for contact lens associated microbial keratitis, *Contact lens anterior eye the journal of the British Contact Lens Association,* 25(1), pp 3-9.

Zhonghua, Yan. Ke. Za. Zhi. (1992), Keratitis associated with contact lens wear. *Chinese Journal of Ophthalmology*, 28(4), pp 234-235. (24)

3

Keratitis Caused by Onchocerciasis: *Wolbachia* Bacteria Play a Key Role

G. Kluxen[1] and A. Hoerauf[2]
[1]*Augenärztliche Überörtliche Gemeinschaftspraxis und Praxisklinik, Wermelskirchen,*
[2]*Institute of Medical Microbiology, Immunlology and Parasitology (IMMIP), University Clinic of Bonn, Bonn, Germany*

1. Introduction

Human beings are the only known important reservoir of *Onchocerca volvulus* which causes onchocerciasis. The adult worms are usually found in subcutaneous nodules and have an average longevity of approximately 15 years. The parasitic worm releases millions of offspring (microfilariae) which migrate through the skin and can enter the anterior or posterior regions of the eye. While alive, the microfilariae appear to cause little or no inflammation, even being in the anterior chamber. However, when they die, either by natural attrition or after chemotherapy, the host response to degenerating worms can result in ocular inflammation (keratitis, uveitis and optic neuritis) that causes progressive loss of vision. Blindness therefore tends to occur in adulthood after many years of infection.

2. Ocular onchocerciasis

The affection starts with a slight conjunctival injection. In Africans an enhancement of the pigmentation at the limbus has also been observed. When phlyctenule-like lesions occasionally appear at the limbus, microfilariae are found in this alteration as well. However, they do not contribute to the development of the keratitis. Here they are only found in a convolution of inflamed cells.

It seems clear that the microfilariae enter the cornea from the limbus via Schlemm's canal and trabeculae (Maertens,1981). The conditions described above, like a slight conjunctival injection, an enhancement of the pigmentation and occasional phlyctenule-like lesions at the limbus indicate the movement of microfilariae in and out of the eye through the conjunctiva.

2.1 Punctate subepithelial stromal keratopathy

The corneal disease typically develops as successive showers of subepithelial lesions on both eyes. The epithelium itself is usually normal and does not stain with either bengal rose or fluorescein. The fluffy opacities („snow flakes", Kératite ponctuée, Keratitis punctata) lie in the superficial layers of the stroma in the interpalpebral region near the limbus (Fig.1) and are accompanied by a considerable amount of photophobia and lacrimation and sometimes by a temporary but slight impairment of visual acuity. They are due to an oedema developing around the dead microfilariae. They may remain for a longer time but eventually resolve without trace, but these lesions tend to develop more and more as long as intracorneal death of the worms continues; and when the keratopathy progress moves on lesions in the deeper stroma occur.

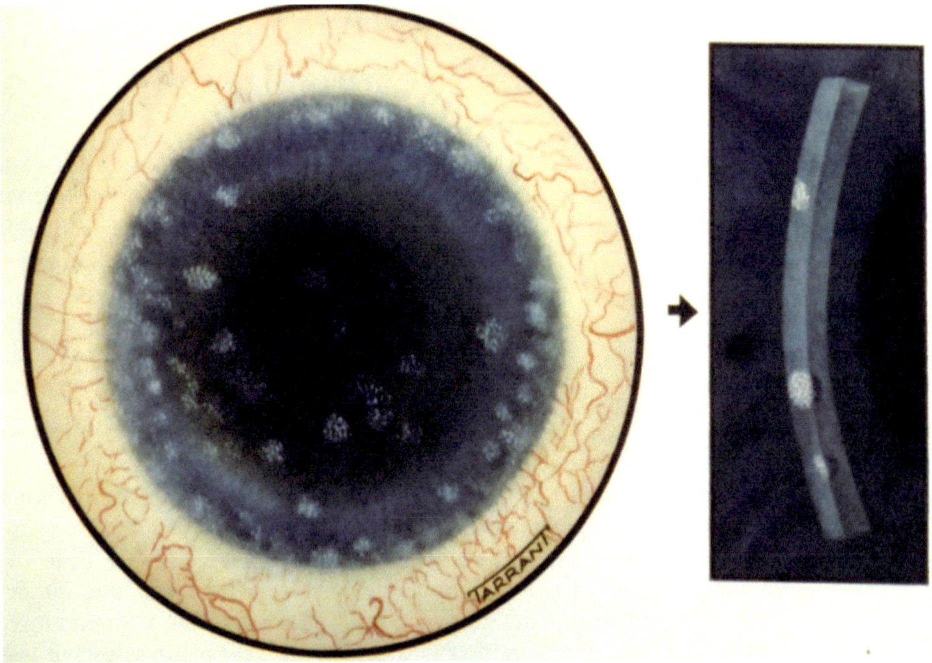

Fig. 1. Well-marked onchocercal keratitis as punctate subepithelial stromal keratopathy in a European, focal section of the cornea showing the punctate infiltration of the anterior subepithelial layers (Choyce, 1958).

Following the terminology of Duke-Elder and Leigh (Duke-Elder, 1965; Duke-Elder & Leigh, 1966) this keratitis is termed: Punctate subepithelial stromal keratopathy (Fig.1). The opacities of subepithelial facet formation appear also as immune response after perforating graft keratoplasty (Pleyer, 1997). An increasingly evident subepithelial keratopathy caused by onchocerciasis with a variation in infiltration size is also called linear keratitis (Keratitis linearis, Kératitis linéaire) and demonstrates the characteristic appearance of "cracked ice" (glace brisée) (Woodruff et al., 1963). The ephithelium of the cornea remains even and transparent for a long time.

Microfilariae in the cornea are predominantly positioned in a horizontal angle along the corneal nerves (Maertens,1981). They remain in this one position for a long time and then move laboriously through the interstitium (stroma) (Fig.2). After the administration of diethylcarbamazine (DEC) microfilariae tend to move into the cornea. They squirm and roll, then die and elongate stretched. At this point a punctate subepithelial stromal keratopathy (keratitis punctate, punctate keratitis) develops (WHO,1982). The dead microfilariae become opaque, decay and then disappear. Over the next few weeks and months the generated opacity of the cornea can either improve, remain as it is or worsen. Histologically there are eosinophil and neutrophil granulocytes around the dead microfilariae in the cornea stroma. The latter ones are attracted by Wolbachia (Saint André et al., 2002; Gentil & Pearlman, 2009).

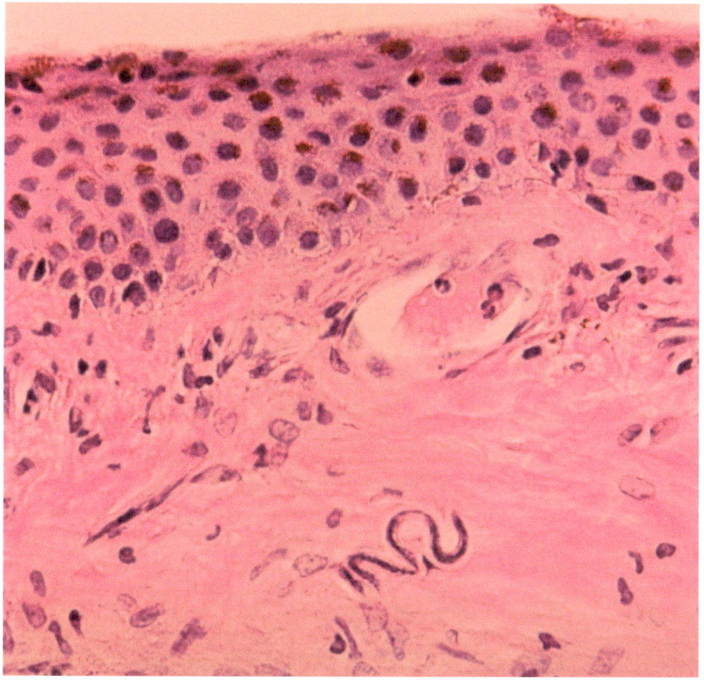

Fig. 2. A microfilaria of *Onchocerca volvulus* in a corneal scar of the stroma, H.E. staining, by courtesy of Hj.Trojan

In Central America cases in this particular phase were already called interstitial keratitis (Branly,1956), while the European authors in Africa used to call a keratopathy only interstitial if minor vascularisation was also present. However, the cornea affected by ocular onchocerciasis partially remains transparent for a long time (Fig.3, Fig.4).

2.2 Band-shaped keratopathy and sclerosing keratitis

The grey opacity is always being separated from the limbus by a clear zone. The limbal edge is sharp while the axial edge slowly fades away, tailing off in scattered spots and cracks. As a general rule of the band-shaped keratopathy the opacity spreads slowly over some years towards the center until the two segments from temporal and nasal meet. However, when a sclerosing keratitis occurs in onchocerciasis it usually evolves from a confluence of several foci of invasion around the lower half of the limbus (Fig.3), typically from tongues between the 3 and 9 o'clock positions, and progresses as an apron round the lower half of the cornea. The upper part with the center of the cornea is at this time initially clear (Fig.4). A few superficial blood vessels, lying at first between the epithelium and Bowman's membrane, invade the cornea. The progress gradually spreads upwards; the invading vessels break through Bowman's membrane and often penetrate into the stroma. In an acute destructive process the keratocytes as well as the fibrillae suffer from necrosis, and in a reparative stage keratocytes multiply and various degenerative changes occur with the development of fibrosis in the stroma, where eosinophils as well are components of the cellular infiltrates, and changes in the overlying epithelium which typically becomes heavily pigmented by the migration of pigmented cells in and from the limbus.

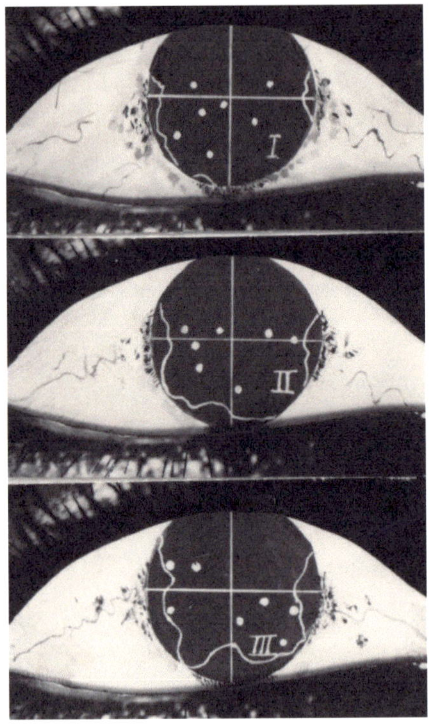

Fig. 3. Development in progress of the sclerosing keratopathy over two years in a young African man with ocular onchocerciasis. The boarder of corneal infiltration from the limbus is shown by the line; the points are larger opacities from punctate subepithelial stromal keratopathy.

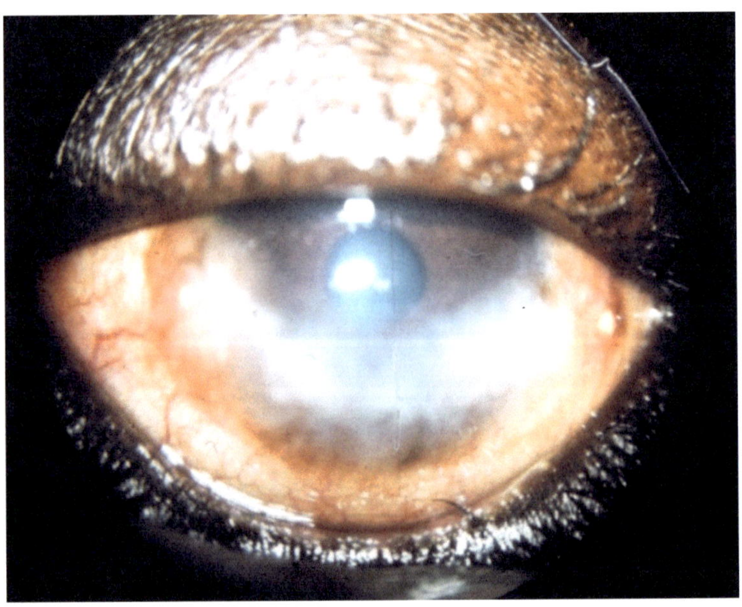

Fig. 4. Keratitis semilunaris, a form of the band-shaped keratopathy, by courtesy of Hj.Trojan

The cornea has thickened by now, has an uneven surface and is no longer transparent (Fig.5, Fig.6). There are callosities (scars, adherences, synechia) in the inside of the eye and a hypotension can foster the development of a phthisis bulbi, a hypertension a staphyloma of the cornea (Fig.6). The affected eye has turned blind irrevocably and usually the process repeats itself almost simultaneously in the other eye. The cases of sclerosing keratitis increase drastically in endemic onchocerciasis regions particularly in affected people above the age of sixty (Rodger & Maertens 1977).

2.3 Discussion of the clinical picture (with differential diagnosis)

2.3.1 Keratitis through onchocerciasis is not an infectious but an inflammatory condition

In ocular onchocerciasis cases the subepithelial opacities in the peripheral cornea initially occur in almost even large patches. They are not a specific pathognomonic indication but are rather an epiphenomenon in a series of infectious eye diseases; they are similar to the facet formations caused by adenovirus- or chlamydia-keratitides (Bialasiewicz & Jahn,1989). However, these keratitides each have their small individual characteristics. They also occur in zoster and varicella with characteristically larger patches, and were further observed in leprosy and avitaminosis (Maertens,1981). The latter diseases are predominantly inflammatory responses, just like the inflammatory reaction after keratoplasty (Preyer, 1997).

A sclerosing keratitis or band-shaped keratopathy is a late complication occurring in all chronic uveitides therefore this condition of the ocular onchocerciasis is not a specific pathognomonic indication. When a sclerosing keratopathy is developing (Fig.5, Fig.6), other major processes adherent to an uveitis have already occurred in the eye since this severe syndrome cannot develop isolated in the cornea. A keratitis caused by onchocerciasis may not be termed infectious, but it is an infestation like ophthalmomyiasis or cysticercosis (Kanski et al., 2005) and is mainly an inflammatory condition.

2.3.2 Subepithelial facet formations occur also in Dimmer's nummular keratitis

Dimmer's nummular keratitis is a slowly-developing benign keratitis without an accompanying conjunctivitis and usually unilaterally, characterized by disc-shaped facet infiltrates in the superficial layers of the corneal stroma. It occurs endogenous in small areas of Central Europe, particularly in Austria, where Friedrich Dimmer [1855-1926] worked (Duke-Elder & Leigh,1965). Sporadic reports about similar cases have come from East Europe and America, China and South Africa. The disease appears among young land-workers and the incidence is seasonal, the peak period being after the harvest in the autumn. The most striking feature is that the opacities occur deep in the parenchyma and mainly central in location.

2.3.4 How pathology develops in onchocerciasis and what is new?

In the anterior segment, microfilariae infiltrate the cornea, where they die as a result of antifilarial therapy or by natural attrition. It was thought that this strong inflammatory reaction after the death of the microfilariae in the eye was probably due to a release of toxins. This is not the fact, but research has identified a major cause (Saint André et al., 2002): *Wolbachia* endosymbionts.

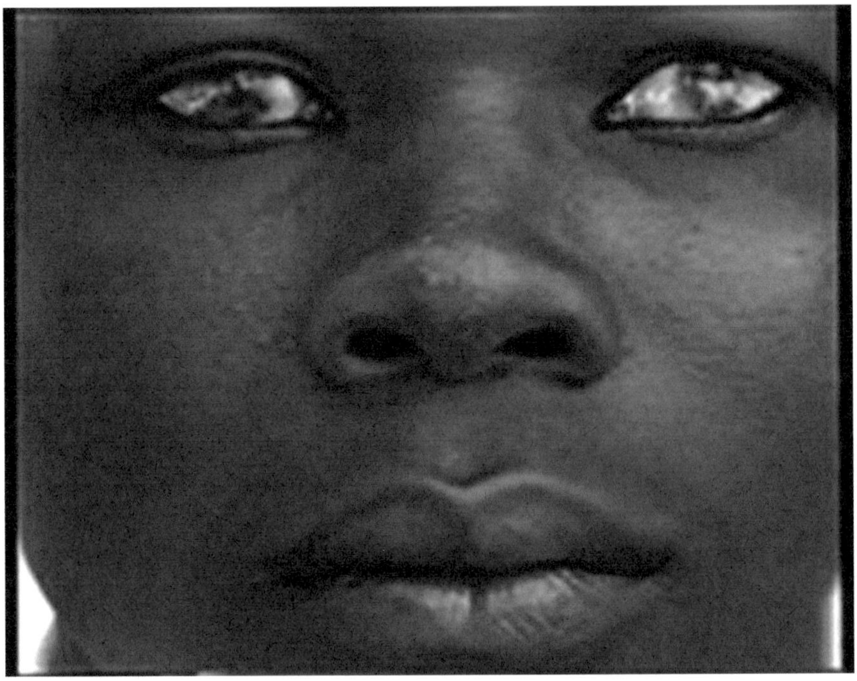

Fig. 5. General view of the corneal opacity, here band-shaped sclerosing keratopathy in a horizontal axis, the young man from Bossangoa is blind with amaurosis.

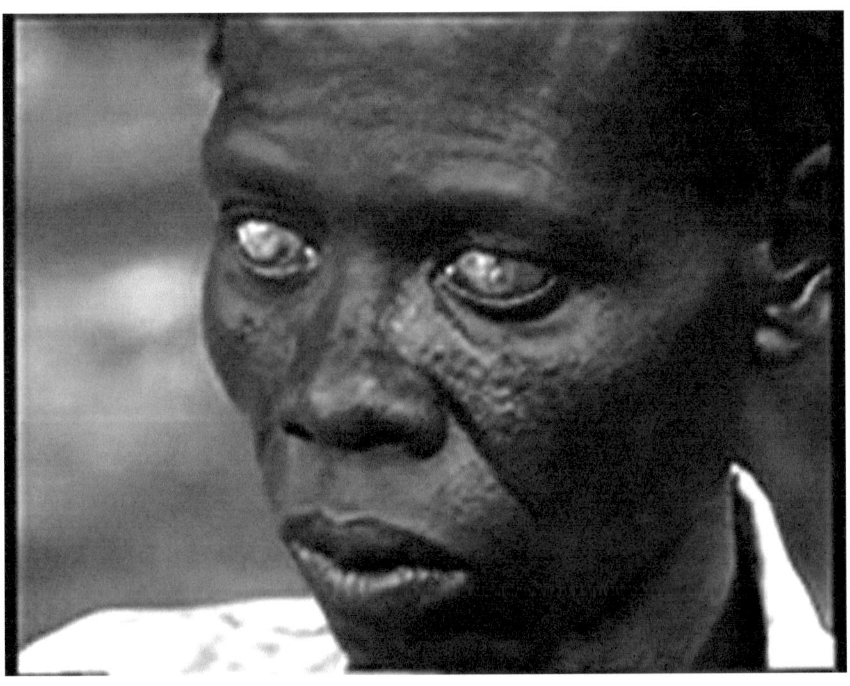

Fig. 6. General view of the corneal opacity, sclerosing keratitis and staphylomata in both sides, amaurosis, man from Bossangoa

3. Prevalence of keratitis caused by onchocerciasis

Knowledge on prevalence and incidence of keratitis through onchocerciasis is limited, and currently there are no surveys available considering the prevalence and incidence of keratitis caused by onchocerciasis in Bossangoa in the North-West of the Central African Republic. In 1994, when the mass-distribution of ivermectin in the area had started, a survey on blindness and visual impairment had been undertaken in this district (Schwartz et al., 1997). The region, with a population of around 100,000, was particularly hyper- and mesoendemicly infected with onchocerciasis. Blindness and visual impairment caused by onchocerciasis was found in 219 cases (bilateral blindness 98, unilateral blindness 49 and visual impairment 72) of 6086 inhabitants. This demonstrates a prevalence of *Onchocerca*-attributable ocular pathology including punctate keratitis of 3.6 %. The major causes for blindness in the region (prevalence of 2.2%) were found to be onchocerciasis (73.1%), cataract (16.4%), trachoma (4.5%), and glaucoma (2.2%). Continuous monitoring of the Bossangoa district was interrupted, because the eye clinic, as well as most of Bossangoa's other buildings, was destroyed in 2002 during the revolution. The eye clinic has been reconstructed since and ophthalmic work is being continued in the town, but it would still be too dangerous to undertake a visit to the district before peace is restored in the area. It remains a conflict area and CDTI (Community directed treatment with Ivermectin) guidelines are never met. A few years after ivermectin therapy had been introduced a decreased number of cases of blindness, mainly attributable to onchocerciasis, had been observed in a comparable community in the North-West sector of the Central African Republic after five years of ivermectin treatment (Kennedy et al., 2002), but there were no changes in the prevalence of main ocular lesions. The mass-distribution of the medication had been interrupted with the outbreak of the conflict. In order to be effective the drug Mectizan® (Ivermectin) must be given to 65 % of all community members for 15-20 years, which correlates with the length of the worm's life cycle.

4. *Wolbachia* endosymbionts

In the worms of *Onchocerca volvulus* endosymbionts (bacteria called *Wolbachia*) are located in a specialized anatomical and physiological microenvironment. In adult filarial worms, *Wolbachia* are mainly found throughout the hypodermal cells of the lateral cords, and are in the embryos and microfilariae. The worm relies on these intracellular living bacteria for its homeostasis. The association between *Wolbachia* and filarial nematodes is obligatory and not parasitic. It is a mutual partnership (Fenn & Blaxter, 2007). The hypodermal lateral cord, where *Wolbachia* are mainly found, may be considered as a special organ for *Wolbachia*. The first appearance of *Wolbachia* in the scientific literature was a description of the bacteria within ovaries of mosquitoes (Hertig,1936; Kozek & Rao, 2007). *Onchocerca volvulus* and other nematodes harbour endosymbiotic *Wolbachia* bacteria throughout their life cycles, and they are passed on to the next generation of worms through the oocyte in a vertical transmission like an inherited strain.

As nematode *Wolbachia* lack factors like genetic selection or recombination, the rapid development of resistance to any drug found to have antiwolbachial activity would be hindered. Data from *Wolbachia* genomes can be used to better understand the biology of these organisms (Pfarr & Hoerauf, 2005). It is easy to work out why this bacteria needs to live inside a cell by looking at genome content. For example, *Wolbachia* of *Brugia malayi* does not have the capacity to synthesise all of the amino acids required for protein synthesis and so must import these from the host cell. On the other hand, the filarial worms themselves are apparently unable to synthesize riboflavins or haem endogenously, but their *Wolbachia* has a full set of genes to provide these important co-factors (Yamada et al., 2007).

4.1 *Wolbachia* play the main role in causing river blindness

It has become increasingly clear that *Wolbachia* play a major role in the pathogenesis of ocular onchocerciasis (river blindness) in the human host. Neutrophil infiltration and development of corneal disease occur only when *Wolbachia* are present (Saint André et al. 2002). Eliminating the endobacteria by doxycycline treatment in infected individuals reduces adverse reactions to current drug therapies and even reduces early stages of pathology (Hoerauf et al., 2000; Hoerauf & Pfarr, 2007).

The development of the pathology in the infected person is now thought to be a hyperimmune response to worm antigens (Hoerauf & Pfarr, 2007). But particularly *Wolbachia* are strong inducers of the immune responses. A reaction from dead worm material (without *Wolbachia*) into contact with the filarial-infected host is the recruitment of surrounding eosinophils and macrophages, infiltrations in the skin and other tissues.

The most striking feature is that *Wolbachia*, these "bugs within the bug", are inherent in some filarial worms that infect man and animals, contribute to severe pathological manifestations of filarial infections, and offer a novel approach to chemotherapy and control of filarial infections, especially onchocerciasis.

4.2 Evidence in favour of the role of *Wolbachia* in the pathogenesis of onchocerciasis

4.2.1 *Wolbachia* contribute to severe pathological manifestations

Human monocytes incubated with *O. volvulus* extracts containing *Wolbachia* stimulated the production of proinflammatory and chemotactic cytokines compared with extracts from *O. volvulus* nodules in the absence of Wolbachia (Brattig et al., 2001). Furthermore, *Wolbachia* are required for recruitment of neutrophils, innate inflammatory cells, to the onchocercomata (skin nodules containing *O. volvulus*), as the number of neutrophils in nodules from doxycycline-treated individuals (Fig.7) is greatly reduced compared with untreated patients (Brattig et al., 2001; Saint André et al.; 2002). Neutrophils are only found surrounding worms which contain *Wolbachia*.

Wolbachia are strong inducers of the immune response. A connection between the very severe filarial pathology in onchocerciasis and *Wolbachia* infection has also been demonstrated by an in vivo model for blindness in mice (Saint André et al., 2002). The development of neutrophil infiltration and development of a corneal haze in mice after injection of worm extract into the cornea is dependent upon the presence of *Wolbachia* as *O. volvulus* extract depleted of *Wolbachia* (Fig.7) does not induce keratitis which is also not induced when these mice do not have a functional Toll-like receptor (TLR) 4 molecule (Hise et al., 2003, Saint André et al., 2002). TLRs are key receptors in the innate immune reaction to foreign antigens. Also TLR 2 plays a role in the development of ocular pathology (Daehnel et al., 2007; Gentil & Pearlman, 2009). Strong candidates and inducers of the immune response are *Wolbachia surface* protein and surface glycolipoproteins/glycolipids (Fenn & Blaxter, 2007).

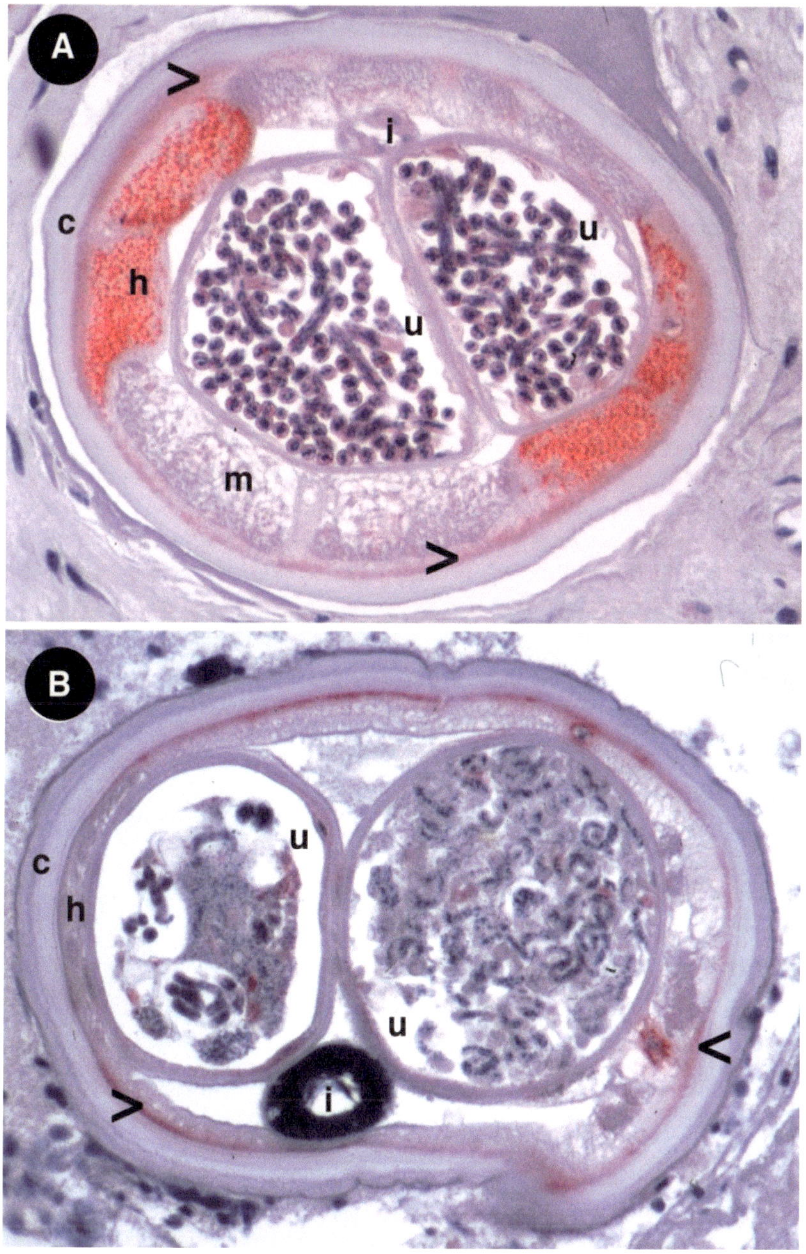

Fig. 7. Immunohistology of midbody cross-sections of female *Onchocerca volvulus* filariae. Staining with rabbit antiserum against bacterial hsp-60 was used. (A) Worm from control: Bacteria are red stained in the hypodermal cords (h) and in the embryos; cuticle (c), musculature (m), intestine (i), uteri (u) show normal embryogenesis with stretched microfilariae: x 180. (B) Worm from patient after doxycycline treatment (ivermectin + doxycycline for 6 weeks, nodulectomy 4 months later): No bacteria are detectable in the hypodermis, a weak staining is shown in areas of mitochondrial density (arrows). Embryos in uteri are degenerated and embryogenesis is interrupted: x 135 (Hoerauf et al., 2000) by courtesy of Elsevier Science.

A recent finding showed that *Wolbachia* numbers are more abundant in *O. volvulus* sampled from infections where severe ocular disease is common, compared to samples from a forested area where blindness is rare (Higazi et al., 2005). In this study, the strain from the savannah shown to cause more severe ocular disease had significantly higher *Wolbachia* loads compared with a less virulent strain from a forested area.

4.2.2 *Wolbachia* contribute to the adverse reactions after microfilaria treatment

Most of the evidence supporting a role for *Wolbachia* in the pathogenesis of filarial diseases stems from posttreatment adverse reactions in infected individuals. For example, systemic treatment of onchocerciasis patients with diethylcarbamazine (DEC) causes rapid death of the microfilariae in the skin and eyes, resulting often severe posttreatment side effect the so called "Mazzotti reaction". The severity of the "Mazzotti reaction" is dependent on the number of microfilariae containing *Wolbachia* in the skin and eyes (Hoerauf & Pfarr, 2007). Reactions include fever, headache, dizziness, myalgia, arthralgia, tachycardia, ciliary injection, severe pruritus and enlargement of lymph nodes. However, this test is absolutely out-mode now. The reactions resemble the >erisipela de la costa< of Guatemala, which also develops during the needling of head-nodules and the killing of adult worms resulting in a severely thickened face (Kluxen, 2011).

4.3 An autoimmological reaction in the retina

Twenty years ago it had been suggested that autoimmunological reactions resulting from cross-reactivity between parasite antigens and components of eye tissues contribute to development of ocular onchocerciasis (Braun et al.,1991). The *Onchocerca volvulus* antigen Ov39 (39 kDa) is cross-reactive with a retinal antigen of 44 kDa and induces ocular inflammation in rats after immunization (McKechnie et al., 2002). This reaction is thought to develop without a contribution of *Wolbachia*.

5. Conclusion

Findings from studies on infected individuals and animal models demonstrate that endosymbiotic *Wolbachia* have a profound effect on the pathogenesis of the disease. Pathology of ocular onchocerciasis starts with the induction of cytokines by macrophages and monocytes dependent on the presence of *Wolbachia*. A potential molecule that is mediating the inflammatory response is Wolbachia surface protein, which elicits a strong inflammatory response via TLR 2 and TLR 4 (Daehnel et al., 2007; Hise et al., 2003; Saint André et al., 2002; Brattig et al., 2004; Gentil & Pearlman, 2009).

The strain of *O. volvulus* shown to cause more severe ocular disease had significantly higher *Wolbachia* loads compared with another, less virulent strain, indicating a correlation between virulence and *Wolbachia* in ocular onchocerciasis (Higazi et al., 2005). One implication may be that *Wolbachia* boosts immune responsiveness toward filarial antigens, facilitating the clearance of microfilariae and the development of immunopathogenesis (Pfarr et al. 2007). The severity of severe posttreatment side effects has been associated with the microfilarial load of the body before treatment and the antihelmintic drug used to kill the microfilariae (Hoerauf & Pfarr, 2007).

It has become increasingly clear that *Wolbachia* play a major role in the pathogenesis of ocular onchocerciasis (river blindness) in the human host. Neutrophil infiltration and development of corneal disease occur only when *Wolbachia* are present (Saint André et al., 2002; Gentil & Pearlman, 2009). However, the presence of *Wolbachia* in filariae should not be considered as being solely responsible for all the pathological manifestation seen in filarial infections as a weak reaction from dead worm material can also be observed.

Wolbachia are an excellent target for the development of new antifilarial drugs because of their essential role in worm embryogenesis, development and adult survival (Hoerauf et al., 2007). Eliminating the endobacteria (Fig.7) reduces adverse reactions to current drug therapies and even reduces early stages of pathology. Preliminary data indicate (Daehnel et al., 2007) that the elimination of the endobacteria from the worms by doxycycline treatment in infected individuals will also limit the severity of punctate keratitis.

The current mainstay of mass treatment by the World Health Organization's African Programme for Onchocerciasis Control (APOC) is ivermectin, an antiparasitic agent that kills microfilariae and inhibits the growth and proliferation of offspring for several months at a time; it targets mature microfilariae. But the treatment with ivermectin does not cure the disease. Ivermectin + doxycycline cause sterility in adult worms and thereby directly suppress the embryonic development of the worm. The dosage of doxycycline was 100 mg/day p.o. for six weeks and the dosage of Mectizan® (ivermectin) was 2 times 150µg/kg during and 4 - 6 months after doxycycline treatment (Hoerauf et al., 2001), and another dosage of 200 mg/day doxycycline for 4 - 6 weeks was sufficient to kill over 60% of the female worms (Hoerauf et al., 2008; Taylor et al., 2010). Studies have shown that the combination of ivermectin and doxycycline significantly enhanced ivermectin-induced suppression of microfilariae, effectively blocking disease transmission for as long as years, possibly irreversibly.

6. References

Bialasiewicz, A.A. & Jahn, G.J. (1989). *Chlamydieninfektionen*, Enke, Stuttgart

Branly, M.A. (1956). Über die Onchozerkosis (Morbus Robles). *Klinische Monatsblätter für Augenheilkunde*, Vol.128, No.1, pp. 1-15

Brattig, N.W.; Büttner, D.W. & Hoerauf, A. (2001): Neutrophil accumulation around *Onchocerca* worms and chemotaxis of neutrophils are dependent on *Wolbachia* endobacteria. *Microbes and Infection*, Vol.3, pp. 439-446

Brattig, N.W.; Bazzocchi, C. & Kirschning, C.J. et al. (2004). The major surface protein of *Wolbachia* endosymbionts in filarial nematodes elicits immune responses through TLR2 and TLR4. *Journal of Immunology*, Vol.173, pp. 437-445

Braun, G.; McKechnie, N.M.; Connor V.; Gilbert, C.E.; Engelbrecht F., Whitworth J.A. & Taylor D.W. (1991). Immunological crossreactivity between a cloned antigen of *Onchocerca volvulus* and a component of the retinal pigment epithelium. *Journal of Experimental Medicine*, Vol.174, (July 1991), pp. 169-177 www.jem.org

Choyce, D.P. (1958). Some observations on the ocular complications of onchocerciasis and their relationship to blindness. *Transactions of the Royal Society of Tropical Medicine and Hygiene*, Vol.52, pp. 112-121

Daehnel, K.; Hise, A.G.; Gillette-Ferguson I.; Pearlman, E. (2007). *Wolbachia* and *Onchocerca volvulus*: Pathogenesis of river blindness, In: A. Hoerauf & R.U. Rao (eds.), *Wolbachia: A bug's life in another bug, Issues in Infectious Diseases*, Vol.5, pp. 133-145, ISBN 978-3-8055-8180-6

Duke-Elder, St. (1965). Diseases of the outer eye. In: Sir St. Duke-Elder (ed.), *System of Ophthalmology*, Kimpton, London, Vol.VIII/1, pp. 401-425, ISBN 0-85313-218-6

Duke-Elder, S. & Leigh, A.G. (1966). Diseases of the outer eye. In: Sir St. Duke-Elder (ed.), *System of Ophthalmology*, Kimpton, London, Vol.VIII/2, pp. 733-751, ISBN 0-85313-218-6

Fenn, K. & Blaxter, M. (2007). Coexist, cooperate and thrive: *Wolbachia* as long-term symbionts of filarial nematodes, In: A. Hoerauf & R.U. Rao (eds.), *Wolbachia: A bug's life in another bug, Issues in Infectious Diseases*, Vol.5, pp. 66-76, ISBN 978-3-8055-8180-6

Gentil, K. & Pearlman, E. (2009). Gamma interferon and interleukin-1 receptor 1 regulate neutrophil recruitment to the corneal stroma in a murine model of Onchocerca volvulus keratitis. *Infection and Immunity*, Vol. 77, No.4 (April 2009), pp. 1606-1612

Hertig, M. (1936). The rickettsia, *Wolbachia pipientis* (Gen. et Sp. Nov.) and associated inclusions of the mosquito, *Culex pipiens*. *Parasitology*, Vol.28, pp. 453-486

Higazi, T.B.; Filiano, A.; Katholi, C.R.; Dadzie, Y.; Remme, J.H. & Unnasch T.R. (2005). *Wolbachia* endosymbiont levels in servere and mild strains of *Onchocerca volvulus*. *Molecular and Biochemical Parasitology*, Vol.141, No.1 (May 2005), pp. 109-112 http://ini.sagepub.com

Hise, A.G.; Gillette-Ferguson, I. & Pearlman, E. (2003). Immunopathogenesis of *Onchocerca volvulus* keratitis (river blindness): a novel role for TLR 4 and endosymbiotic *Wolbachia* bacteria. *Journal of Endotoxin Research*, Vol.9, No.6, pp. 390-394 www.sciencedirect.com

Hoerauf, A.; Volkmann, L.; Hamelmann, C.; Adjei, O.; Autenrieth, I.B.; Fleischer, B. & Büttner, D.W. (2000). Endosymbiotic bacteria in worms as targets for a novel chemotherapy in filariasis. *The Lancet*, Vol.355, No.9211 (April 2000), pp. 1242-1243

Hoerauf, A.; Mand, S.; Adjei, O.; Fleischer, B. & Büttner, D.W. (2001). Depletion of *Wolbachia* endobacteria in *Onchocerca volvulus* by doxycycline and microfilaridermia after ivermectin treatment. *The Lancet*, Vol.357, No. 9266 (May 2001), pp. 1415-1416

Hoerauf, A. & Pfarr, K. (2007). *Wolbachia* Endosymbionts: An Achilles' heel of filarial nematodes. In: A. Hoerauf & R.U. Rao (eds.), *Wolbachia: A bug's life in another bug. Issues in Infectious Diseases*, Vol.5, pp. 31-51, ISBN 978-3-8055-8180-6

Hoerauf, A.; Specht, M.; Büttner, M.; Pfarr, K., Mand, S. et al. (2008). *Wolbachia* endobacteria depletion by doxycycline as antifilarial therapy has macrofilaridical activity in onchocerciasis: a randomized placebo-controlled study. *Medical Microbiology and Immunology*, Vol.197, No.3 (September 2008), pp. 295-311

Kanski, J.J.; Milewski, S.A.; Damato, B.E.; Tannar, V. (2005). *Diseases of the ocular fundus*. Elsevier Mosby, ISBN 0-723433704, Edinburgh

Kennedy, M.H.; Bertocchi, A.D.; Hopkins, A.D.; Meredith, S.E. (2002). The effect of 5 years of annual treatment with ivermectin (Mectizan®) on the prevalence and morbidity of onchocerciasis in the village of Gami in the Central African Republic. *Annals of Tropical Medicine and Parasitology*, Vol.96, No.3, pp. 297-307

Kluxen, G. (2011). *Dr. Jean Hissette's research expeditions to elucidate river blindness.* Kaden, ISBN: 978-3-922777-99-1, Heidelberg

Kozek, W.J. & Rao, R.U. (2007). The discovery of *Wolbachia* in arthropods and nematodes - a historical perspective. In: A. Hoerauf & R.U. Rao (eds.), *Wolbachia: A bug's life in another bug. Issues in Infectious Diseases*, Vol.5, pp. 1-14, ISBN 978-3-8055-8180-6

Maertens, K. (1981). Les complications oculaires de l'Onchocercose. *Annales de la Société Belge de Médecine Tropicale*, Vol.61, pp. 199-224

McKechnie, N.M.; Gürr, W.; Yamada, H., Copland, D. & Braun, G. (2002). Antigen mimicry: *Onchocerca volvulus* antigen-specific T cells and ocular Inflammation. *Investigative Ophthalmology & Visual Science,* Vol.43, No.2 (February 2002), pp. 411-418 www.iovs.org

Pfarr, K. & Hoerauf, A. (2005). The annotated genome of *Wolbachia* from the filarial nematode *Brugia malayi*: What it means for progress in antifilarial medicine. *PLoS Medicine*, Vol.2, No.4 (April 2005), pp. 0283-0286 www.plosmedicine.org

Pfarr, K.; Foster, J. & Slatko B. (2007). It takes two: Lessons from the first nematode *Wolbachia* genome sequence, In: A. Hoerauf & R.U. Rao (eds.), *Wolbachia: A bug's life in another bug. Issues in Infectious Diseases*, Vol.5, pp. 52-65, ISBN 978-3-8055-8180-6

Pleyer, U. (1997). Immunreaktion nach perforierender Keratoplastik. Immunbiologie, Prävention und Therapie. *Der Ophthalmologe*, Vol.94, pp. 933-950

Rodger, F.C. & Maertens, K. (1977). Ophthalmology. In: F.C. Rodger (ed.), *Onchocerciasis in Zaire. A new approach to the problem of river blindness*, Pergamon Press, Oxford U.K., chapter 6, pp. 105-130

Saint André, A.v.; Blackwell, N.M.; Hall L.R.; Hoerauf, A. et al. (2002). The role of endosymbiotic *Wolbachia* bacteria in the pathogenesis of river blindness. *Science*, Vol.295, (March 2002), pp. 1892-1895 www.sciencemag.org

Schwartz, E.C.; Huss, R.; Hopkins, A.; Dadjim, B.; Madijitoloum, P.; Hénault, C. & Klauss, V. (1997). Blindness and visual impairment in a region endemic for onchocerciasis in the Central African Republic. *British Journal of Ophthalmology*, Vol.81, No.7 (July 2002), pp. 443-447

Taylor, M.J.; Hoerauf, A. & Bockarie, M. (2010). Lymphatic filariasis and onchocerciasis. *The Lancet*, Vol.376, No. 9747 (October 2010), pp. 1175-1185

WHO expert group (1982). Pathogénie et traitement de l'onchocercose oculaire : Rapport de la huitième réunion du groupe scientifique de travail « filariose » en collaboration avec le programme de prévention de la cécité. *Issue of the World Health Organization*, WHO/TDR/FIL/SWG (8)/82.3 (unpublished document, contains the collective views of an international group of experts: Maertens, K.; Thylefors, B.; Zéa-Flores, G.; Dadzié, Y.; Duke, B.O.L.; Rolland, A.; Taylor, H.R.; Donnelly, J.J.; Nussenblatt, R. & Ottesen, E.A.)

Woodruff, A.W.; Barnley, G.R.; Hooland J.T.; Jones D.E.; McCrae A.W.R.; McLaren D.S. (1963). Onchocerciasis and the eye in Western Uganda. *Transactions of the Royal Society of Tropical Medicine and Hygiene*, Vol.57, (January 1963), pp. 50-63

Yamada, R.; Brownlie, J.C.; McGraw, E.A. & O'Neill, S.L. (2007). Insights into *Wolbachia* biology provided through genomic analysis, In: A. Hoerauf & R.U. Rao (eds.), *Wolbachia: A bug's life in another bug. Issues in Infectious Diseases*, Vol.5, pp. 77-89, ISBN 978-3-8055-8180-6

4

Corneal Collagen Cross-Linking Using Riboflavin and Ultraviolet-A Irradiation in Keratitis Treatment

Vassilios Kozobolis, Maria Gkika and Georgios Labiris
Eye Institute of Thrace and Department of Ophthalmology, Medical School of Democritus University of Thrace
Greece

1. Introduction

Cross-linking is a common method of tissue stabilization. For example, cross-linking is used for formaldehyde-induced tissue stiffening and fixation in pathologic specimens. Corneal collagen Crosslinking (CXL) is performed with ultraviolet-A (UVA) irradiation at 370 nm and the photosensitizer riboflavin (vitamin B_2). According to Wollensak (Wollensak, 2006), the photosensitizer is excited into its triplet state generating reactive oxygen species (ROS), which are mainly singlet oxygen and to a much lesser degree superoxide anion radicals. ROS can react further with various molecules inducing chemical covalent bonds that form bridges between amino groups of collagen fibrils (type II photochemical reaction). The biomechanical effect occurs immediately after irradiation leading to an increase of the biomechanical rigidity of the cornea of about 300%. The optimal wavelength of the ultraviolet (UV) radiation is 370 nm, at which riboflavin presents maximal absorption. Interestingly, a similar mechanism has been detected in the human crystalline lens (Krishna et al., 1991).

2. Corneal collagen cross-linking therapeutic protocol

All patients who are candidates for CXL treatment need to have maximum keratometric (K) readings less than 60 diopters (D) and a central corneal thickness (CCT) of at least 400 μm. All clinical trials of CXL refer to patients aged between 18 and 30 years. There are as yet no extensive clinical trials in children and this is the reason why great care must be taken when applying the CXL technique in patients younger than 18. In addition, patients with a history of herpetic keratitis, corneal scarring, severe eye dryness, pregnancy or nursing, previous anterior segment surgery, systemic collagen pathology or concomitant autoimmune diseases should be handled with great caution and perhaps better excluded.

In brief, the CXL procedure is conducted under sterile conditions in the operating room, after the patient's eye is anesthetized. According to the Dresden therapeutic protocol, the central 8 mm of the corneal epithelium are removed to allow better diffusion of riboflavin into the stroma. Without epithelial removal, the biomechanical effect is less than 50% of the standard cross-linking procedure. In fact, Botto´s et al. (Botto´s et al., 2008) conclude in their study that treatment of the cornea with riboflavin and UVA without previous de-epithelialization did not induce any cross-linking effect. Consequently, to facilitate diffusion of riboflavin throughout the corneal stroma, the epithelium should be removed as an important initial step in the treatment (Botto´s et al., 2008). Partial grid-pattern epithelial removal allows some riboflavin penetration, but uptake is limited and non-homogeneous, which may affect the efficacy of the cross-linking process (Samaras et al., 2009). Following de-epithelialization, a 0.1% riboflavin solution (10 mg riboflavin-5-phosphate in 10 ml dextran 20% solution) is instilled to the cornea for 30 min (2 drops every 2 min) prior to the irradiation, until the stroma is completely penetrated and the aqueous humour is stained yellow. Changes in application time and riboflavin concentration have only little influence on stromal depth diffusion (Søndergaard et al., 2010). Generally, the riboflavin film is an integral part of the CXL procedure and important in achieving the correct stromal and endothelial UVA irradiance (Wollensak et al., 2010). The irradiation is performed from 1 cm distance for 30 min using a UVA double diode at 370 nm and an irradiance of 3 mW/cm^2 (equal to a dose of 5.4 J/cm^2). The required irradiance is controlled in each patient directly before the treatment to avoid a potentially dangerous UVA overdose (Wollensak et al., 2003a, 2003b). Instillation of riboflavin drops (1 drop every 2 min) is continued during irradiation as well, in order to sustain the necessary concentration of riboflavin. Moreover, balanced salt solution (BSS) is applied every 6 min to moisten the cornea.

A series of variations of the treatment protocol have been demonstrated. In 2009 Kanelopoulos (Kanellopoulos, 2009) demonstrated that CXL by means of a femtosecond laser facilitated intrastromal 0.1% riboflavin administration, with promising preliminary results. A limited but favourable effect of trans-epithelial CXL was noted on keratoconic eyes, without complications by Leccisotti et al. (Lecciotti and Islam, 2010). The effect appears to be less pronounced than described in the literature after CXL with de-epithelialization. In addition Bakke et al. (Bakke et al., 2009) attempted to compare the severity of postoperative pain and the rate of penetration of riboflavin between eyes treated by CXL using excimer laser superficial epithelial removal and mechanical full-thickness epithelial removal, and concluded that superficial epithelial removal using the excimer laser resulted in more postoperative pain and the need for prolonged application of riboflavin to achieve corneal saturation.

3. Laboratory studies

A series of laboratory studies attempted to explore all aspects of CXL procedure and particularly its biomechanical, thermomechanical, and morphological impact on corneal cells. A series of observations suggest that the CXL effect is maximal on the anterior part of cornea, the collagen fibre diameter is significantly increased only in the anterior half of the stroma, in enucleated porcine eyes CXL led to a significant change in the swelling behaviour of the anterior stroma (Wollensak et al., 2007a) and significant biomechanical and biochemical differences between the anterior and posterior parts were demonstrated in post-CXL corneas (Kohlhaas et al., 2006; Schilde et al. 2008).

Microcomputer-controlled biomaterial testing experiments indicated an impressive increase in corneal rigidity of 71.9% in porcine and 328.9% in human corneas, and an increase in Young's modulus by a factor of 1.8 in porcine and 4.5 in human corneas after CXL. Moreover, clinical observations suggest that riboflavin/UVA-induced collagen cross-linking leads to an increase in biomechanical rigidity which remains stable over time (Wollensak and Iomdina, 2009; Kling et al., 2010).

However, the cross-linking effect was maximal only in the anterior 300 μm. The greater biomechanical effect in human corneas was attributed to the relatively larger portion of crosslinked stroma because of the lower total corneal thickness of 550 μm in human corneas compared with 850 μm in porcine corneas (Wollensak et al., 2003c). Also, in a patient with acute keratoconus (KC) who underwent CXL, a rapid progress of KC developed 2 years after treatment. This was probably due to the fact that CXL does not effectively treat the posterior corneal layers and Descemet's membrane, which are mainly affected by acute KC. In normal corneas, the anterior stroma is more rigid because it is designed to maintain the anterior corneal curvature. Interestingly, the anterior stroma of these corneas after CXL is found to be more cross-linked and still more rigid than the posterior one. This degree of rigidity is even preserved in the presence of corneal oedema (Muller et al., 2002).

In the anterior stroma of rabbit corneas treated with CXL, the collagen fibre diameter was significantly increased by 12.2% (3.96 nm), but by only 4.6% (1.63 nm) in the posterior stroma (Wollensak et al., 2004c). Similar changes have been reported in the cornea and other tissues due to age-related or diabetes mellitus-related collagen cross-linking. A possible explanation for this observation is that the induced cross-links push the collagen polypeptide chains apart, resulting in increased intermolecular spacing. On scanning electron microscopy, the collagen fibres of cross-linked vitreous humour also appeared markedly thickened and coarse (Faulborn et al., 1998).

Experiments in rabbits treated with riboflavin and variable UVA irradiances ranging from 0.75 to 4 mW/cm^2 indicated a variable apoptosis that was proportional to the irradiance power. The cytotoxic UVA irradiance level for keratocytes was determined to be about 0.5 mW/cm^2 (Wollensak et al., 2004a). The latter was also confirmed by in vitro studies on keratocyte cell cultures (Wollensak et al., 2004b). Cytotoxic apoptosis is followed by repopulation approximately after 4–6 weeks from the irradiation (Wollensak at al., 2007b).

In addition, in cross-linked porcine eyes, a markedly increased resistance to collagenase digestion was described, with a 15 day digestion time in the cross-linked samples compared with 6 days in the controls (Spoerl et al., 2004). This effect is stronger in the anterior half of the cornea.

4. Corneal collagen cross-linking in keratitis

Corneal ocular infections may have a profound and devastating impact on visual function. Ulcerative keratitis, often microbial in origin and presenting as central or peripheral corneal ulceration or infiltration, is a sight-threatening condition. It remains an important cause of blindness that requires skilled management and effective chemotherapy to preserve vision (Bennett et al., 1998). If diagnosis and initiation of appropriate antimicrobial treatment are delayed, it has been estimated that only 50% of eyes will heal with good visual outcome (Jones et al., 1981)

Although the treatment of corneal infections with topical antimicrobial agents has been notably successful, with an expanding array of both focused and broad-spectrum antibiotics, there has been an alarming resistance to antimicrobial agents (Neu, 1992; DeMuri and

Hostetter, 1995; Dever, 1996; Glynn et al., 1998; Levy, 1998). Microbes cleverly develop resistance to antibiotics as a result of chromosomal mutation, inductive expression of a latent chromosomal genes, or exchange of genetic material via transformation, bacteriophage transduction, or plasmid conjugation (Neu, 1992; Bennett et al., 1998). Use of the fluoroquinolones in the management of external infections is the most recent example of how a new class of antibiotics has been instrumental in changing management strategies for the treatment of corneal infections. Also, the antimicrobials currently in use are sometimes problematic because of their toxic effects on the ocular surface (e.g., punctate keratitis, delayed re-epithelialization, hyperemia, chemosis). Nonetheless, emerging patterns of resistance even to these new classes of antimicrobial agents (Daum et al., 1990; Smith et al., 1990; Thomson et al., 1991; Snyder et al. 1992; Maffett et al. 1993; Chin and Marx, 1994; Fass et al., 1995; Knauf et al., 1996; Garg et al., 1999; Goldstein et al., 1999) have stimulated the continuing quest for an agent that provides rapid and complete microbicidal activity with minimal toxic effects and susceptibility to mechanisms of microbial resistance.

The antimicrobial activity of UV irradiation includes sporicidal and virucidal effects. Traditional applications of UV light are disinfection of drinking water and air/surface disinfection. Limitations of the application of UV are mainly the lack of penetration and a strong dependence on the distance from the UV source, which may result in non-homogeneous microbial inactivation.

On the other hand, riboflavin, or vitamin B2, is a naturally occurring compound and an essential human nutrient. Riboflavin products, including lumichrome, are present and consumed in a wide range of foods and natural products in common use. Japanese scientists demonstrated in the 1960s that riboflavin, when exposed to visible or UV light, could be used to inactivate the RNA containing tobacco mosaic virus (Tsugita et al., 1965) Research has been developing since 2000 to use riboflavin as a photosensitizer to inactivate pathogens in plasma, platelet, and red cell products (Goodrich, 2000). The chemistry, toxicity, and ability of riboflavin to interact with nucleic acids after UVA photograph activation have also been extensively studied. Riboflavin and UVA (280-370 nm) may damage nucleic acids by direct electron transfer, production of singlet oxygen, and generation of hydrogen peroxide with formation of hydroxyl radicals. Pathogen DNA/RNA may be affected in the absence of oxygen. This process has proven effective against a wide range of pathogens, including bacteria, intracellular HIV-1, West Nile virus (WNV), and porcine parvovirus in preclinical studies of platelets and plasma. The process also damages leukocyte DNA in a manner that makes repair by normal pathways unlikely. There is a possibility that the riboflavin already present in the cornea serves as a natural antimicrobial mechanism. However, riboflavin concentration in the cornea is not enough to produce antimicrobial effects in overt keratitis. Since the riboflavin is photosensitive, it is more likely that the small content of corneal riboflavin will be depleted when exposed to sunlight UVA/riboflavin therefore may offer high efficacy with low protein damage and little toxicity.

This development leads to propose that it could act as a photosensitizer useful for the inactivation of pathogens found in corneal infections, because of its nucleic acid specificity and its limited tendency toward indiscriminate oxidation. Pitts et al. (Pitts et al., 1977) found corneal damage at the surface UVA dose (365 mV) of 42.5 J/cm2, and Wollensak et al. (Wollensak et al., 2004a) described that riboflavin/UVA treatment leads to dose-dependent keratocytes damage in human corneas. The recent clinical use of a riboflavin/UVA combination for corneal collagen cross-linking and the observations in the laboratory of keratocyte depletion after its application (Wollensak et al., 2003a, 2003b; Labetoulle, 2003; Kaufman, 2004) stimulated the evaluation of its application for corneal infection and the effort ultimately to expand the armamentarium of antimicrobial agents for the management of severe keratitis.

4.1 Corneal collagen cross-linking in infectious keratitis

In 2008, Martins et al. (Martins et al., 2008) demonstrated the antimicrobial properties of CXL against common pathogens. Some of the microbes used in this study were selected from a panel of human clinical ocular isolates from severe cases of bacterial keratitis treated at The Wilmer Ophthalmological Institute and maintained by the Microbiology Laboratory, Johns Hopkins University School of Medicine. The test panel of human clinical isolates maintained by the previously mentioned mcrobiology laboratory included oxacillin-resistant Staphylococcus epidermidis (ORSE), penicillin-resistant Streptococcus pneumoniae (PRSP), and pan-resistant Pseudomonas aeruginosa (PRPA). The other isolates used were individual cultures of freeze-dried microorganisms used to assist in the quality control of microbiologic media (LyfoCults; PML Microbiologicals, Wilsonville, OR), which included ORSE strain (SE), methicillin-resistant Staphylococcus aureus (MRSA), oxacillinsusceptible Staphylococcus aureus (SA), and susceptible Pseudomonas aeruginosa (PA). Candida albicans (CA) strains were selected from human clinical isolates in the Virology Sector and maintained bythe Microbiology Laboratory (Johns Hopkins University School of Medicine). Approximately 90% of cases of bacterial keratitis is caused by one of four groups of organisms (1): PA (2) SA and Micrococcaceae, (3) SP, and (4) Enterobacteriaceae (Jones, 1979) Pseudomonas keratitis is one of the most serious corneal infections and represents one of the most threatening bacterial infections of the eye. Because of its aggressive behaviour and the frequency and context in which it occurs, PA was chosen as a pathogen in this study. SA was also used because of its frequency of occurrence as a clinical pathogen. SE is an uncommon clinical corneal pathogen; however, its common presence at the ocular surface and its occasional conversion to an opportunist led to its selection as a comparison test organism. SP is commonly associated with keratitis (3%–15% of cases).

They tested the riboflavin/UVA combined treatment against two settings of organisms based on their antibiotic susceptibility. Group 1 comprised non-resistant organisms: SA, PA, and SE. Group 2 was formed by antibiotic-resistant organisms: MRSA, PRPA, PRSP. CA was also tested in the same settings. The assay used was a disc diffusion susceptibility test based on the principle that a standardized inoculum of the organism is swabbed onto the surface of a Mueller-Hinton agar plate, and filter paper discs (Kirby-Bauer discs) impregnated with antimicrobial agents are placed on the agar. In this study, the discs were placed in the culture plates as reference points, to locate the areas were the riboflavin was previously instilled. The discs were also taken as a guide measurement for planimetric assays. Riboflavin drops were placed directly adjacent to the discs, to have an area where the light exposure would be performed. After 20 minutes of diffusion of the drops in the agar media, a beam of UVA light was directed to the selected location for 1 hour, in an attempt to photoactivate the vitamin solution or simply to irradiate the area of bacterial growth with UVA alone. The experiments were performed three times for each microorganism. After UVA irradiation, the agar plates were inverted and incubated for 24 hours at 34°C to 35°C in an ambient-air incubator Digital images of each disc and the surrounding agar area were captured (AxioVision software; Axiovert 200M; Carl Zeiss Meditec Inc., Thornwood, NY), to measure the area of inhibition zone to the nearest whole millimetre (Herretes et al., 2006). The mean growth inhibition zone (GIZ) in square millimeters is inversely proportional to the minimum inhibitory concentration (MIC) of the organisms.

The results in the present study showed significant in vitro inhibition growth of test isolates using UVA alone and combined riboflavin/UVA treatment compared with the other types of treatment used in the study (B2 alone and B2 previously activated by UVA), for both setting of microorganisms. Seemingly, the results also demonstrate that UVA treatment alone is less effective in killing test isolates when compared with riboflavin/UVA combined treatment in the groups of bacteria tested. Of interest, a very localized response to the area of irradiation was observed, with well-defined margins of bactericidal activity, which may be particularly useful for corneal application. Riboflavin alone did not seem to have any effect as an antibacterial agent, but UVA alone may be effective against all test isolates in this study but resistant PA. The combined riboflavin/UVA treatment did not seem to have any effect on CA at the riboflavin concentrations tested (0.1% and 0.5%). In the non-resistant group, the efficacy of riboflavin/UVA treatment was greater against SA and SE, when compared with the treatment applied against PA. In the resistant group, we found the same effect, with the treatment being more effective against the Gram-positive microorganisms than against PA. Despite those findings, we cannot exclude PA as a potential microorganism to be treated with riboflavin/UVA treatment, as it showed some GIZ in both groups.

In 2010 Sauer et al. (Sauer et al., 2010) demonstrated the antimicrobial properties of riboflavin/UVA (365 nm) against fungal pathogens. The antimicrobial properties of riboflavin/UVA (365nm), with or without previous treatment with amphotericin B, were tested on three groups of fungi selected from severe cases of keratomycosis: *Candida albicans*, *Fusarium* sp, and *Aspergillus fumigatus*. They were tested by using Kirby-Bauer discs with empty disc (control), riboflavin 0.1% alone (R), UVA alone (UVA), riboflavin 0.1% and additional UV-A exposure (R_UVA), amphotericin B alone (A), amphotericin B and riboflavin 0.1% (A_R), amphotericin B and UVA (A_UVA), amphotericin B and riboflavin 0.1%, and additional UVA exposure (A_R_UVA). The mean growth inhibition zone (GIZ) was measured around the discs. *C. albicans*, *Fusarium* sp, and *A. fumigatus* did not show any increased GIZ after treatment without previous amphotericin B medication. However, GIZ was significantly greater after pretreatment with amphotericin B and riboflavin/UVA (A_R_UVA) for *C. albicans* (P=.0005), *Fusarium* sp (P=.0023) and *A. fumigatus* (P=.0008) compared with A, A_R, and A_UV-A. Amphotericin B is believed to interact with fungi membrane sterols to produce aggregates that form transmembrane channels. Given that collagen is one of the principal components of the cornea, it is also probable that amphotericin B may diffuse easily after cross-linking. Previous treatment with amphotericin B allowed riboflavin/UVA effectiveness against *C. albicans*, *Fusarium* sp, and *A. fumigatus*. This schema might be used in the future for the treatment of keratomycosis.

Since these results obtained in vitro do not always correlate with in vivo efficacy, further tissue culture models and animal studies are under way to test the efficacy of this treatment for infectious keratitis. Iseli et al. (Iseli et al., 2008) evaluated the efficacy of CXL for treating infectious melting keratitis. Five patients with infectious keratitis associated with corneal melting were treated with CXL when the infection did not respond to systemic and topical antibiotic therapy. Follow-up after cross-linking ranged from 1 to 9 months. In all cases, the progression of corneal melting was halted after CXL treatment. Emergency keratoplasty was not necessary in any of the five cases presented. Moreover, Micelli-Ferrari et al. (Micelli-Ferrari et al., 2009) described a case of keratitis caused by the Gram-negative Escherichia coli treated with CXL with outstanding outcome. Similar results were also reported by More´n et al. (More´n et al., 2010), who treated an infectious keratitis using CXL.

4.2 Corneal collagen cross-linking in complicated bullous keratopathy with ulcerative keratitis

CXL's antimicrobial and anti-oedematous properties were demonstrated by (Kozobolis et al., 2010) in our report of two patients with combined bullous keratopathy and ulcerative keratitis, resistant to conventional treatments. Former investigators suggested that corneal cross-linking (CXL) might have beneficial impact against corneal melting from bacterial and fungal enzymes, because of the antimicrobial effect of UV-A radiation per se (Spoerl et al., 2004). Moreover, there is evidence that the post-CXL corneal stabilization might prevent the outflow of aqueous humour to the intracorneal space in diseases that manifest with endothelial decompensation. Based on the aforementioned hypothesis and evidence, we reported our experience with 2 patients with bullous keratopathy and corneal infectious keratitis resistant to topical medical treatment who underwent therapeutic CXL.

The first patient was a 78-year-old woman referred to our department because of deteriorating visual acuity (VA) and intense ocular discomfort (pain) in the right eye, whereas her left eye was otherwise healthy. Regarding the ophthalmological history, she had an extracapsular cataract extraction surgery in her right eye 4 years before her referral. According to her medical report, because of high postoperative intraocular pressure, she was administered timolol–dorsolamide. fixed combination (twice a day). The systemic history revealed diabetes and coronary heart disease. Ophthalmological examination revealed the following: A vision-threatening central corneal ulcer accompanied by bullous keratopathy (Figurel), which resulted in poor visualization of the anterior chamber structures (Figure 2). Despite limited visibility, an anterior chamber intraocular lens could be visualized, in situ. Best-corrected visual acuity (BCVA) was limited to light perception, whereas corneal thickness (thinnest point) measured by ultrasound pachymetry (Pacline Optikon pachymeter, Optikon 2000 SpA; OPTIKON, Rome, Italy) was 641 mm (Table 1). The second patient was a 69-year-old man referred to our department because of deteriorating VA and intense ocular discomfort (pain) in his left eye, whereas his right eye was otherwise healthy. Regarding the ophthalmological history, he had an extracapsular cataract extraction surgery in his left eye, 3 years before his referral. Ever since the cataract operation, the patient was administered dorsolamide–timolol fixed combination because of postoperative ocular hypertension. His systemic history was uneventful. BCVA was 1/20 (Table 1). Slit-lamp biomicroscopy revealed bullous keratopathy accompanied by infectious keratitis (Figure 3). The corneal thickness at the thinnest point was 714 mm (Table 1). Further to antiglaucoma medications, both patients were administered intense local antibiotic treatment (ofloxacin and tobramycin drops). However, their private physicians reported progressive deterioration of the bullous keratopathy and depth of their ulcers. Because of the vision-threatening state of their corneas and the poor beneficial effect of local antibiotics, CXL was suggested as an experimental but potentially vision-saving adjuvant treatment.

The same surgical procedure was applied to both patients, according to the Dresden protocol. Prior antibiotic therapy was resumed after the surgical procedure with the addition of frequent instillation of artificial tears. Patients' progress was monitored in a daily basis for the first postoperative week for thorough evaluation of the reepithelialization process and potential adverse events and then every 15 days for a total of 2-month follow-up period.

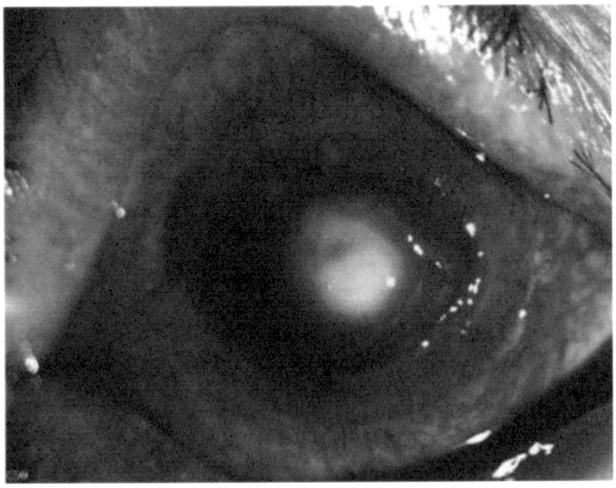

Fig. 1. Preoperative picture (case 1).

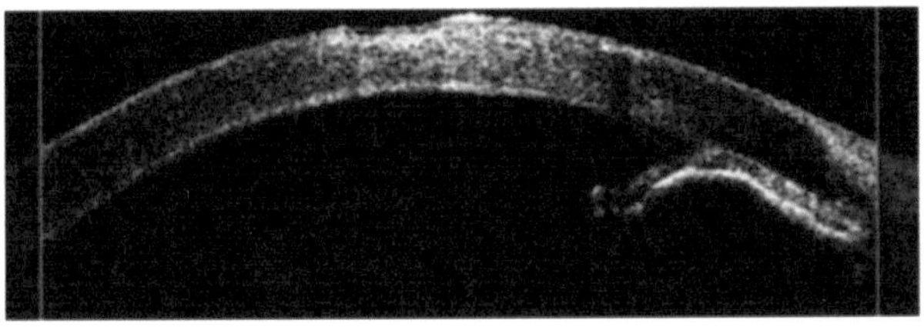

Fig. 2. Preoperative anterior chamber optical coherence tomography (case 1).

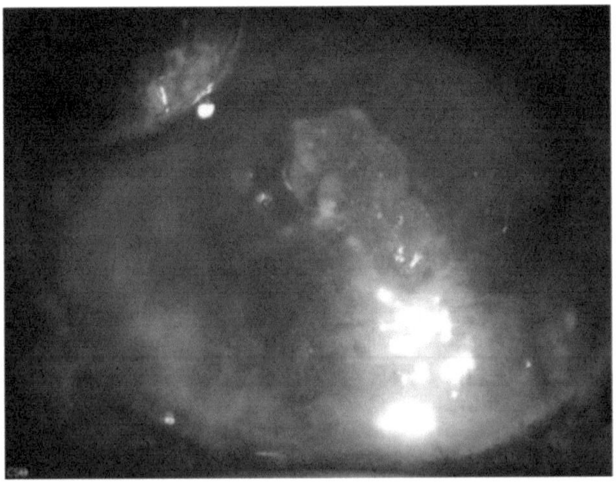

Fig. 3. Preoperative picture (case 2).

Both patients presented a gradual reduction of their corneal edemas associated with improved corneal clarity and VA. Moreover, slit-lamp biomicroscopy revealed significant improvement of the corneal ulcers (Table 1, Figures 4-7). The reepithelialization was completed within a week for both cases. Laboratory analysis of the corneal epithelial smears was negative in the first case, whereas in the case 2, Streptococcus viridans was developed. BCVA was improved in both cases within the first month after the treatment and remained stable during the follow-up period of 2 months.

	Preoperative		Postoperative	
	VA (Decimal Scale)	Corneal Thickness (Thinnest Point) (μm)	VA (Decimal Scale)	Corneal Thickness (Thinnest Point) (μm)
Case 1, 78-year-old woman	LP	641	2/10	595
Case 2, 68-year-old man	1/20	714	2/10	635

LP, light perception.

Table 1. Preoperative and Postoperative VA and Corneal Thickness

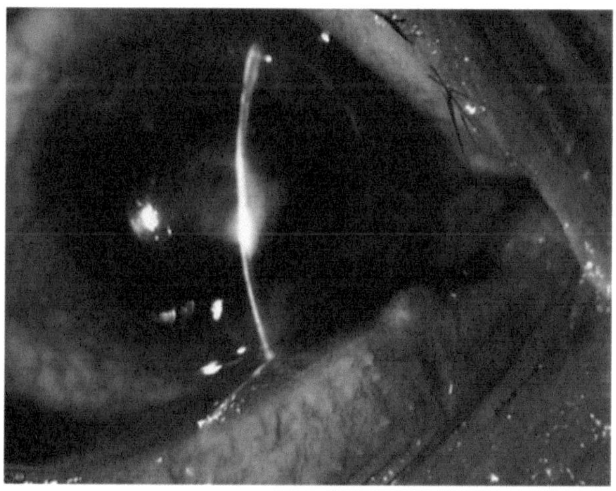

Fig. 4. First postoperative day (case 1).

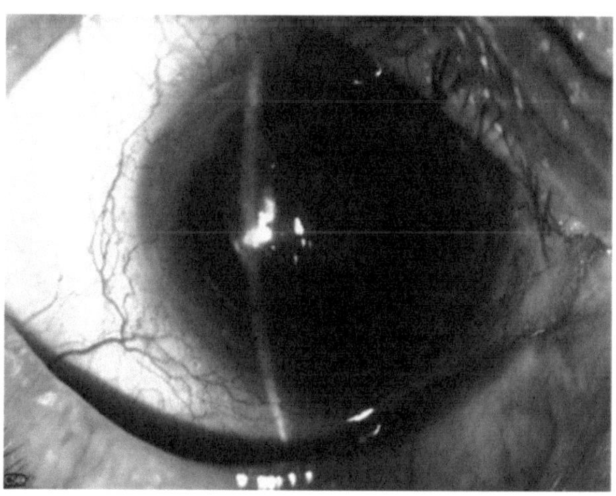

Fig. 5. Final postoperative day (case 1).

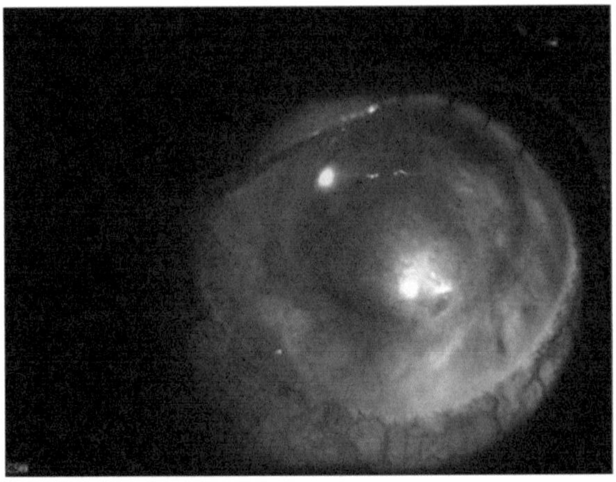

Fig. 6. First postoperative day (case 2).

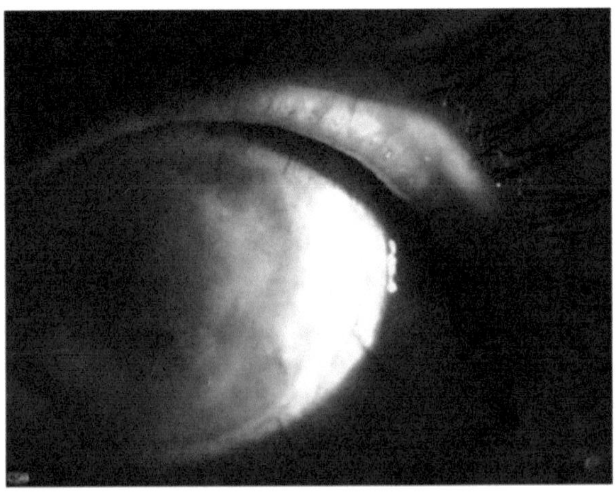

Fig. 7. Final postoperative day (case 2).

Regarding the cases presented above, the induced compactness of the cornea after CXL treatment interfered with the outflow of aqueous humor to the intracorneal space because of the decompensated endothelium. In fact, the impact of riboflavin and UV radiation on endothelial decompensation has been also described by Ehlers et al. (Ehlers et al., 2009). Our results confirm their hypothesis because both patients presented a decrease of their corneal thickness and disappearance of the corneal bullae. Moreover, the beneficial impact of the CXL treatment on corneal edema because of endothelial dysfunction might be inversely related to the extent of dysfunction. Thus, maximal therapeutic results are expected in early stages of endothelial decompensation. These results attempt to contribute to the body of knowledge regarding the potential therapeutic use of CXL with riboflavin in patients with bullous keratopathy and corneal infectious keratitis resistant to topical medical treatment that would otherwise be treated with penetrating keratoplasty. Obviously, more studies are required to explore the potential beneficial impact of the proposed therapeutic procedure and provide the necessary data for the development of a valid therapeutic protocol.

5. Risks and side-effects

Riboflavin is generally regarded as a safe compound since it is a vitamin ingested in normal diets and an omnipresent molecule in biological systems. It is also assumed that any residual riboflavin and any photoproducts produced during the treatment do not present any hazardous risks.

On the other hand, UV represents a potential danger to the human eye. It is well known that UV-induced photochemical damage, like sunburn or photokeratitis, is caused by UVB light, wavelengths of 270 to 315 nm, at power densities ranging from 0.12 to 0.56 J/cm^2. In the cornea UVB light (290–320 nm) is mainly absorbed by the corneal epithelium (Pitts et al., 1977; Podskochy, 2004). CXL uses a small peak-like sector of the UVA spectrum (370 nm). UVA absorption in the cornea is increased massively during the cross-linking procedure due to the photosensitizer riboflavin, resulting in a UVA transmission of only 7% across the cornea (Wollensak et al., 2003a). Experiments in rabbits indicated that the cytotoxic level for the corneal endothelium was 0.36 mW/cm^2. The standard CXL procedure cannot provide this cytotoxic level unless the central corneal thickness (CCT) is less than 400 µm (Wollensak et al., 2003d, 2003e). In general, UVA is absorbed mainly by the crystalline lens, which also contains endogenous riboflavin and other photosensitizers leading to cross-linking of crystallines (Krishna et al., 1991). This intrinsic system protects the retina and for this reason a UV absorber is usually incorporated into intraocular lenses. For the development of cataract, various power values have been reported in the literature at wavelengths between 290 and 365 nm.(Pitt s et al., 1977; Olsen et al., 1982; Soderberg et al., 2003; Wollensak et al., 2004a; Kumar et al., 2004; Lin et al., 2004;) With the standard CXL procedure, the lens only receives 0.65 J/cm^2 which is far below the cataractogenous level of 70 J/cm^2 (Pitts et al., 1977). The retina is damaged by thermal or visible-light-induced photochemical damage in the wavelength range of 400–1400 nm. In the rhesus monkey, retinal damage with complete loss of the photoreceptor layer was reported at a threshold level of 81 mW/cm^2; however, such extreme values are incompatible with the standard treatment protocol (Zuclich, 1989).

On the other hand, after CXL, the stroma is depopulated of keratocytes. HRT II-RCM confocal microscopy indicated that the reduction in anterior and intermediate stromal keratocytes is followed by gradual repopulation which will be concluded within 6 months. The UVA induces oxygen radicals which in turn induce covalent cross-linking of all kinds of proteins. The main and almost exclusive protein of the cornea is collagen type I, so that in the cornea the effect is focused on collagen. UVA can induce DNA and RNA lesions, an effect which is used for the disinfection of water etc. and also for the sterilization of aphaeresis blood products, efficiently killing viruses, bacteria and other pathogens. These cytotoxic DNA lesions are also the reason for the cytotoxic effect of the treatment on corneal keratocytes. As long as the cornea treated has a minimum thickness of 400 µm (as recommended), the corneal endothelium will not experience damage, nor will deeper structures such as lens and retina. The light source should provide a homogenous irradiance, avoiding hot spots (Mazzotta et al., 2007a; 70Spoerl et al., 2007; Avitabile et al., 1997; Mencucci et al. 2010; Esquenazi et al., 2010). Nevertheless, Mazzotta et al. (Mazzotta et al., 2007b) presented two cases, studied through in vivo confocal microscopy, with stage III KC that developed stromal haze after the cross-linking treatment, Kymionis et al. (Kymionis et al., 2010) reported the development of posterior linear stromal haze after simultaneous PRK followed by CXL and Raiskup et al. (Raiskup et al., 2009), after an extensive one-year study of 163 eyes, concluded that advanced KC should be considered at higher risk of haze development after CXL due to low corneal thickness and high corneal curvature. In addition, Koppen et al. (Koppen et al., 2009) reported four cases of keratitis and corneal scarring from a total of 117 eyes treated with CXL and Sharma et al. (Sharma et al., 2010) presented a case report of Pseudomonas keratitis after collagen cross-linking for KC. Also, Garcia-Delpech et al. (Garcia-Delpech et al., 2010) reposted a case of Fusarium keratitis 3 weeks after healed corneal cross-linking. Apart from the above-mentioned complications, Gokhale et al. (Gokhale and Vemuganti, 2010) presented a case of acute corneal melt with perforation in a patient with KC after collagen cross-linking treatment and the use of topical diclofenac and proparacaine eyedrops. The use of diclofenac sodium and proparacaine eyedrops after surgery was possibly responsible for the corneal melt in this patient, so patients who have undergone cross-linking treatment should be observed closely until the corneal epithelium heals completely. In addition, a case of advancing KC treated with CXL complicated with sterile infiltrates was presented by Mangioris et al. (Mangioris et al., 2010). This complication may be an individual hypersensitivity reaction to the riboflavin or UVA light in the anterior stroma. At this point we should mention that Goldich et al. (Goldich et al., 2010) reported that CXL does not cause damage to the corneal endothelium and central retina and Koller et al. (Koller et al. 2009) made a significant effort to evaluate the complication rate of CXL for primary keratectasia and to develop recommendations for avoiding complications. Their results indicate that changing the inclusion criteria may significantly reduce the complications and failures of CXL. A preoperative maximum K reading of less than 58 D may reduce the failure rate to less than 3%, and restricting patient age to younger than 35 years may reduce the complication rate to 1%.

6. Conclusion

CXL is a promising therapeutic intervention for corneal tissue stabilization in diseases that manifest with progressive keratectasia, like keratoconus. Moreover, CXL's anti-oedematous and antimicrobial properties have been demonstrated in a series of studies, suggesting its therapeutic indications in bullous keratopathy and in infectious keratitis, as an adjuvant treatment to conventional therapeutic modalities. These cases show the positive effects of CXL with a satisfactory final visual outcome. CXL may be a promising new treatment for keratitis, although this remains to be elucidated in detail in future studies. Until more data are available this treatment should only be considered in therapy-refractive keratitis or ulceration and not in the first line of defence, since it may have cytotoxic side-effects.

7. References

Avitabile, T., Marano, F., Uva, M.G. & Reibaldi, A. (1997). Evaluation of central and peripheral corneal thickness with ultrasound biomicroscopy in normal and keratoconic eyes. *Cornea* Vol. 16, No. 6, (November 1997), pp. 639–644, ISSN: 02773740

Bakke, E.F., Stojanovic, A., Chen, X. & Drolsum, L. (2009). Penetration of riboflavin and postoperative pain in corneal collagen crosslinking: excimer laser superficial versus mechanical full-thickness epithelial removal. *J Cataract Refract Surg* Vol. 35, No. 8, (August 2009), pp. 1363–1366, ISSN: 08863350

Bennett, H.G.B., Hay, J., Devonshire, P., Kirkness, C.M. & Seal, D.V. (1998). Antimicrobial management of presumed microbial keratitis: guidelines for treatment of central and peripheral ulcers. *Br J Ophthalmol.* Vol. 82, No. 2, (February 1998), pp. 137-145, ISSN: 00071161

Botto´s, K.M., Dreyfuss, J.L., Regatieri, C.V. et al (2008). Immunofluorescence confocal microscopy of porcine corneas following collagen cross-linking treatment with riboflavin and ultraviolet A. *J Refract Surg* Vol. 24, No. 7, (September 2008), pp. S715–S719, ISSN: 1081597X

Chin, G.J. & Marx, Je. (1994). Resistance to antibiotics. *Science* Vol. 264, No. 5157, (1994), pp. 359, ISSN 00368075

Cohen, M.A. & Huband, M.D. (1999). Activity of clinafloxacin, trovafloxacin, quinupristin/dalfopristin, and other antimicrobial agents versus Staphylococcus aureus isolates with reduced susceptibility to vancomycin. *Diagn Microbiol Infect Dis.* Vol. 33, No. 1, (January 1999), pp. 43-46, ISSN: 07328893

Daum, T.E., Schaberg, D.R., Terpenning, M.S., et al. (1990). Increasing resistance of Staphylococcus aureus to ciprofloxacin. *Antimicrob Agents Chemother.* Vol. 34, No. 9, (1990), pp. 1862-1863, ISSN: 00664804

DeMuri, GP & Hostetter, M.K. (1995). Resistance to antifungal agents. *Pediatr Clin North Am.* Vol. 42, No. 3, (1995), pp. 665-685, ISSN: 00313955

Dever, L.L. & Handwerger, S. (1996). Persistence of vancomycin-resistant Enterococcus faecium gastrointestinal tract colonization in antibiotictreated mice. *Microb Drug Resist.* Vol. 2, No. 4, (1996), pp. 415-421, ISSN: 10766294

Ehlers, N., Hjortdal, J., Nielsen, K. & Søndergaard, A. (2009). Riboflavin-UVA treatment in the management of edema and nonhealing ulcers of the cornea. *J Refract Surg* Vol. 25, No. 9, (September 2009), pp. S803–S806, ISSN: 1081597X

Esquenazi, S., He, J., Li, N. & Bazan, HE. (2010). Immunofluoresence of rabbit corneas after collagen cross-linking treatment with riboflavin and ultraviolet A. *Cornea* Vol. 29, No. 4, (April 2010), pp. 412–417 ISSN: 02773740

Fass, R.J., Barnishan, J. & Ayers, L.W. (1995). Emergence of bacterial resistance to imipenem and ciprofloxacin in a university hospital. *J Antimicrob Chemother.* Vol. 36, No. 2, (1995), pp. 343-353, ISSN: 03057453

Faulborn, J., Dunker, S. & Bowald, S. (1998). Diabetic vitreopathy: findings using the celloidin embedding technique. *Ophthalmologica* Vol. 212, No. 6, (1998), pp. 369–376, ISSN: 00303755

Garcia-Delpech, S., Díaz-Llopis, M., Udaondo, P. & Salom, D. (2010). Fusarium keratitis 3 weeks after healed corneal cross-linking. *J Refract Surg.* Vol. 26, No. 12, (December 2010), pp. 994-995, ISSN: 1081597X

Garg, P., Sharma, S. & Rao, G.N. (1999). Ciprofloxacin-resistant Pseudomonas keratitis. *Ophthalmology.* Vol. 106, No. 7, (July 1999), pp. 1319-1323, ISSN: 01616420

Glynn, M.K., Bopp, C., Dewitt, W., et al. (1998). Emergence of multidrug-resistant Salmonella enterica serotype typhimurium DT104 infections in the United States. *N Engl J Med.* Vol. 338, No. 19, (May 1998), pp. 1333-1338, ISSN: 00284793

Gokhale, N.S. & Vemuganti, G.K. (2010). Diclofenac-induced acute corneal melt after collagen crosslinking for keratoconus. *Cornea* Vol. 29, No. 1, (January 2010), pp. 117–119, ISSN: 02773740

Goldich, Y., Marcovich, A.L., Barkana, Y., Avni, I. & Zadok, D. (2010). Safety of corneal collagen cross-linking with UV-A and riboflavin in progressive keratoconus. *Cornea* Vol. 29, No. 4, (April 2010), pp. 409–411, ISSN: 02773740

Goldstein, M.H., Kowalski, R.P. & Gordon, Y.J. (1999). Emerging fluoroquinolone resistance in bacterial keratitis: a 5-year review. *Ophthalmology.* Vol. 106, No. 7, (July 1999), pp. 1313-1318, ISSN: 01616420

Goodrich, R.P. (2000). The use of riboflavin for inactivation of pathogens in blood products. *Vox Sang.* Vol. 78, No. 2, (2000), pp. 211-215, ISSN: 00429007

Herretes, S., Suwan-Apichon, O., Pirouzmanesh, A., et al. (2006). Use of topical human amniotic fluid in the treatment of acute ocular alkali injuries in mice. *Am J Ophthalmol.* Vol. 142, No. 2, (August 2006), pp. 271-278, ISSN: 00029394

Iseli, H.P., Thiel, A.M., Hafezi, F. et al (2008). Ultraviolet A/riboflavin corneal cross-linking for infectious keratitis associated with corneal melts. *Cornea* Vol. 27, No. 5, (June 2008), pp. 590–594, ISSN: 02773740

Jones, D.B. (1979). Initial therapy of suspected microbial corneal ulcers. II. Specific antibiotic therapy based on corneal smears. *Surv Ophthalmol.* Vol. 24, No. 2, (1979), pp. 97-116, ISSN: 00396257

Jones, D.B. (1981). Decision-making in the management of microbial keratitis. *Ophthalmology.* Vol. 88, No. 8, (1981), pp. 814-820, ISSN: 01616420

Kanellopoulos, A.J, (2009). Collagen cross-linking in early keratoconus with riboflavin in a femtosecond laser-created pocket: initial clinical results. *J Refract Surg* Vol. 25, No. 11, (November 2009), pp. 1034–1037, ISSN: 1081597X

Kaufman, H.E. (2004). Strengthening the cornea. *Cornea* Vol. 23, No. 5, (July 2004), pp. 432, ISSN: 02773740

Kling, S., Remon L., Perez-Escudero, A., Merayo-Lloves, J. & Marcos, S. (2010). Corneal biomechanical changes after collagen cross-linking from porcine eye inflation experiments. *Invest Ophthalmol Vis Sci* Vol. 51, No. 8, (August 2010), pp. 3961–3968, ISSN: 01460404

Knauf, H.P., Silvany, R., Southern, P.M.J., et al. (1996). Susceptibility of corneal and conjunctival pathogens to ciprofloxacin. *Cornea.* Vol. 15, No.1, (1996), pp. 66-71, ISSN: 02773740

Kohlhaas, M., Spoerl, E., Schilde, T. et al (2006). Biomechanical evidence of the distribution of cross-links in corneas treated with riboflavin, ultraviolet A light. *J Cataract Refract Surg* Vol. 32, No. 2, (February 2006), pp. 279–283, ISSN: 08863350

Koller, T., Mrochen, M. & Seiler, T. (2009). Complication and failure rates after corneal crosslinking. *J Cataract Refract Surg* Vol. 35, No. 8, (August 2009), pp. 1358–1362, ISSN: 08863350

Koppen, C., Vryghem, J.C., Gobin, L. & Tassignon, M.J. (2009). Keratitis and corneal scarring after UVA/riboflavin cross-linking for keratoconus. *J Refract Surg* Vol. 25, No. 9, (September 2009), pp. S819–S823, ISSN: 1081597X

Kozobolis, V., Labiris, G., Gkika, M., Sideroudi, H., Kaloghianni, E., Papadopoulou, D. & Toufexis, G. (2010). UVA collagen cross linking treatment of bullous keratopathy combined with corneal ulcer. *Cornea* Vol. 29, No. 2, (February 2010), pp. 235–238, ISSN: 02773740

Krishna, C.M., Uppuluri, S., Riesz, P. et al (1991). A study of the photodynamic efficiencies of some eye lens constituents. *Photochem Photobiol* Vol. 54, No. 1, (July 1991), pp. 51–58, ISSN: 00318655

Kumar, V., Lockerbie, O., Kell, S.D. et al. (2004). Riboflavin and UV light based pathogen reduction: extend and consequence of DNA damage at molecular level. *Photochem Photobiol.* Vol. 80, No. 1, (July 2004), pp. 15-21, ISSN: 00318655

Kymionis, G.D., Portaliou, D.M., Diakonis, V.F., Kontadakis, G.A., Krasia, M.S., Papadiamantis, A.G., Coskunseven & E., Pallikaris, A. (2010). Posterior linear stromal haze formation after simultaneous photorefractive keratectomy followed by corneal collagen cross linking. *Invest Ophthalmol Vis Sci* Vol. 51, No. 10, (October 2010), pp. 5030–5033, ISSN: 01460404

Labetoulle, M. (2003). An alternative to corneal transplantation in keratoconus treatment? *J Fr Ophtalmol* Vol. 26, No. 10, (December 2003), pp. 1097–1098 ISSN: 01815512

Leccisotti, A. & Islam, T. (2010). Transepithelial corneal collagen cross-linking in keratoconus. *J Refract Surg* Vol. 26, No. 12, (December 2010), pp. 942–948, ISSN: 1081597X

Levy, S.B. (1998). Multidrug resistance: a sign of the times. *N Engl J Med.* Vol. 338, No. 19, (May 1998), pp. 1376-1377, ISSN: 00284793

Lin, L., Dikeman, R., Molini, B., et al. (2004). Photochemical treatment of platelet concentrates with amotosalen and long-wavelength ultraviolet light inactivates a broad spectrum of pathogenic bacteria. *Transfusion.* Vol. 44, No. 10, (October 2004), pp. 1496-1504, ISSN: 00411132

Maffett, M. & O'Day, D.M. (1993). Ciprofloxacin-resistant bacterial keratitis (letter). *Am J Ophthalmol.* Vol. 115, No. 4, (1993), pp. 545-546, ISSN: 00029394

Mangioris, G.F., Papadopoulou, D.N., Balidis, M.O., Poulas, J.L., Papadopoulos, N.T. & Seiler, T. (2010). Corneal infiltrates after corneal collagen cross-linking. *J Refract Surg* Vol. 26, No. 8, (August 2010), pp. 609-611, ISSN: 1081597X

Martins, S.A., Combs, J.C., Noguera, G. et al (2008). Antimicrobial efficacy of riboflavin/UVA combination (365 nm) in vitro for bacterial and fungal isolates: a potential new treatment for infectious keratitis. *Invest Ophthalmol Vis Sci* Vol. 49, No. 8, (August 2008), pp. 3402–3408, ISSN: 01460404

Mazzotta, C., Balestrazzi, A., Traversi, C. et al (2007a). Treatment of progressive keratoconus by riboflavin-UVA-induced cross-linking of corneal collagen: ultrastructural analysis by Heidelberg retinal tomograph II in vivo confocal microscopy in humans. *Cornea* Vol. 26, No. 4, (May 2007), pp. 390–397, ISSN: 02773740

Mazzotta, C., Balestrazzi, A., Baiocchi, S., Traversi, C. & Caporossi, A. (2007b). Stromal haze after combined riboflavin- UVA corneal collagen cross-linking in keratoconus: in vivo confocal microscopic evaluation. *Clin Exp Ophthalmol* Vol. 35, No. 6, (August 2007), pp. 580–582, ISSN: 14426404

Mencucci, R., Marini, M., Paladini, I., Sarchielli, E., Sgambati, E., Menchini, U. & Vannelli, G.B. (2010). Effects of riboflavin/UVA corneal cross-linking on keratocytes and collagen fibres in human cornea. *Clin Exp Ophthalmol* Vol. 38, No. 1, (January 2010), pp. 49–56, ISSN: 14426404

Micelli-Ferrari, T., Leozappa, M., Lorusso, M. et al (2009). Escherichia coli keratitis treated with ultraviolet A/riboflavin corneal cross-linking: a case report. *Eur J Ophthalmol* Vol. 19, No. 2, (2009), pp. 295–297, ISSN: 11206721

More´n, H., Malmsjo, M., Mortensen, J. & Ohrstrom, A. (2010). Riboflavin and ultraviolet a collagen crosslinking of the cornea for the treatment of keratitis. *Cornea* Vol. 29, No. 1, (January 2010), pp. 102–104, ISSN: 02773740

Muller, L.J., Pels, E. & Vrensen, G. (2002). The specific architecture of the anterior stroma accounts for maintenance of corneal curvature. *Br J Ophthalmol* Vol. 85, (2002), pp. 437–443, ISSN: 00071161

Neu, H.C. (1992). The crisis in antibiotic resistance. *Science* Vol. 257, No. 5073, (1992), pp. 1064-1073, ISSN: 00368075

Olsen, E.G. & Ringvold, A. (1982). Human cornea endothelium and ultraviolet radiation. *Acta Ophthalmol (Copenh).* Vol. 60, No. 1, (1982), pp. 54-56, ISSN: 0001639X

Pitts, D.G., Cullen, A.P. & Hacker, P.D. (1977). Ocular effects of ultraviolet radiation from 295–365 nm. *Invest Ophthalmol Vis Sci* Vol. 16, No. 10, (1977), pp. 932–939, ISSN: 01460404

Podskochy, A. (2004). Protective role of corneal epithelium against ultraviolet radiation damage. *Acta Ophthalmol Scand* Vol. 82, No. 6, (December 2004), pp. 714–717, ISSN: 13953907

Raiskup, F., Hoyer, A. & Spoerl, E. (2009). Permanent corneal haze after riboflavin-UVA-induced cross-linking in keratoconus. *J Refract Surg* Vol. 25, No. 9, (September 2009), pp. S824–S828, ISSN: 1081597X

Samaras, K., O'brart, D.P., Doutch, J. et al (2009). Effect of epithelial retention and removal on riboflavin absorption in porcine corneas. *J Refract Surg* Vol. 25, No. 9, (September 2009), pp. 771–775, ISSN: 1081597X

Sauer, A., Letscher-Bru, V., Speeg-Schatz, C., Touboul, D., Colin, J., Candolfi, E. & Bourcier, T. (2010). In vitro efficacy of antifungal treatment using riboflavin/UV-A (365 nm) combination and amphotericin B. *Invest Ophthalmol Vis Sci.* Vol. 51, No. 8, (August 2010), pp. 3950-3953, 01460404

Schilde, T., Kohlhaas, M., Spoerl, E. & Pillunat, L.E. (2008). Enzymatic evidence of the depth dependence of stiffening on riboflavin/UVA treated corneas. *Ophthalmologe* Vol. 105, No. 2, (February 2008), pp. 165–169, ISSN: 0941293X

Sharma, N., Maharana, P., Singh, G. & Titiyal, J.S. (2010). Pseudomonas keratitis after collagen crosslinking for keratoconus: case report and review of literature. *J Cataract Refract Surg* Vol. 36, No.3, (March 2010), pp. 517–520, ISSN: 08863350

Smith, S.M., Eng, R.H.K., Bais, P., et al. (1990). Epidemiology of ciprofloxacin resistance among patients with methicillin-resistant Staphylococcus aureus. *J Antimicrob Chemother.* Vol. 26, No. 4, pp. 567-572, ISSN: 03057453

Snyder, M.E. & Katz, H.R. (1992). Ciprofloxacin-resistant bacterial keratitis. *Am J Ophthalmol.* Vol. 114, No. 3, (1992), pp. 336-338, ISSN: 00029394

Soderberg, P.G., Michael, R., Merriam, J.C. (2003). Maximum acceptable dose of ultraviolet radiation: a safety limit for cataract. *Acta Ophthalmol Scand.* Vol. 81, No. 2, (April 2003), pp. 165-169, ISSN: 13953907

Søndergaard, A.P., Hjortdal, J., Breitenbach, T. & Ivarsen, A. (2010). Corneal distribution of riboflavin prior to collagen cross-linking. *Curr Eye Res* Vol. 35, No. 2, (February 2010), pp. 116–121, ISSN: 02713683

Spoerl, E., Wollensak, G. & Seiler, T. (2004). Increased resistance of crosslinked cornea against enzymatic digestion. *Curr Eye Res* Vol. 29, No. 1, (July 2004), pp. 35–40, ISSN: 02713683

Spoerl, E., Mrochen, M., Sliney, D. et al (2007). Safety of UVA-riboflavin cross-linking of the cornea. *Cornea* Vol. 26, No. 4, (May 2007), pp. 385–389, ISSN: 02773740

Thomson, K.S., Sanders, C.C. & Hayden, M.E. (1991). In vitro studies with 5 quinolones: evidence for changes in relative potency as quinolone resistance rises. *Antimicrob Agents Chemother.* Vol. 35, No. 11, (1991), pp. 2329-2334, ISSN: 00664804

Tsugita, A., Okada, Y. & Uchara, K. (1965). Photosensitized inactivation of ribonucleic acids in the presence of riboflavin. *Biochim Biophys Acta.* Vol. 103, No. 2, (June 1965), pp. 360-363, ISSN: 00052787

Wollensak, G., Sporl, E. & Seiler, T. (2003a). Treatment of keratoconus by collagen crosslinking. *Ophthalmologe* Vol. 100, No. 1, (January 2003), pp. 44–49, ISSN: 0941293X

Wollensak, G., Spoerl, E. & Seiler, T. (2003b). Riboflavin/ultraviolet- A-induced collagen crosslinking for the treatment of keratoconus. *Am J Ophthalmol* Vol. 135, No. 5, (May 2003), pp. 620–627, ISSN: 00029394

Wollensak, G., Spoerl, E. & Seiler, T. (2003c). Stress–strain measurements of human and porcine corneas after riboflavin– ultraviolet-A-induced cross-linking. J *Cat Refr Surg* Vol. 29, No. 9, (September 2003), pp. 1780–1785, ISSN: 08863350

Wollensak, G., Spoerl, E., Wilsch, M. & Seiler, T. (2003d). Endothelial cell damage after riboflavin-ultraviolet-A treatment in the rabbit. *J Cataract Refract Surg* Vol. 29, No. 9, (September 2003), pp. 1786–1790, ISSN: 08863350

Wollensak, G., Sporl, E., Reber, F. et al (2003e). Corneal endothelial cytotoxicity of riboflavin/UVA treatment in vitro. *Ophthalmic Res* Vol. 35, No. 6, (2003), pp. 324–328, ISSN: 00303747

Wollensak, G., Spoerl, E., Wilsch, M. & Seiler, T. (2004a). Keratocyte apoptosis after corneal collagen cross-linking using riboflavin/UVA treatment. *Cornea* Vol. 23, No. 1, (January 2004), pp. 43–49, ISSN: 02773740

Wollensak, G., Spoerl, E., Reber, F. & Seiler, T. (2004b). Keratocyte cytotoxicity of riboflavin/UVA-treatment in vitro. *Eye* Vol. 18, No. 7, (July 2004), pp. 718–722, ISSN: 0950222X

Wollensak G, Wilsch M, Spoerl, E. & Seiler, T. (2004c). Collagen fiber diameter in the rabbit cornea after collagen crosslinking by riboflavin/UVA. *Cornea* Vol. 23, No. 5, (July 2004), pp. 503–507, ISSN: 02773740

Wollensak, G. (2006). Crosslinking treatment of progressive keratoconus: new hope. *Curr Opin Ophthalmol* Vol. 17, No. 4, (August 2006), pp. 356–360, ISSN: 10408738

Wollensak, G., Aurich, H., Pham, D.T. & Wirbelauer, C. (2007a). Hydration behavior of porcine cornea crosslinked with riboflavin and ultraviolet A. *J Cataract Refract Surg* Vol. 33, No. 3, (March 2007), pp. 516–521, ISSN: 08863350

Wollensak, G., Iomdina, E., Dittert, D.D. & Herbst, H. (2007b). Wound healing in the rabbit cornea after corneal collagen cross-linking with riboflavin and UVA. *Cornea* Vol. 26, No. 5, (June 2007), pp. 600–605, ISSN: 02773740

Wollensak, G. & Iomdina, E. (2009). Long-term biomechanical properties of rabbit cornea after photodynamic collagen crosslinking. *Acta Ophthalmol* Vol. 87, No. 1, (February 2009), pp. 48–51, ISSN: 1755375X

Wollensak, G., Aurich, H., Wirbelauer, C. & Sel, S. (2010). Significance of the riboflavin film in corneal collagen crosslinking. *J Cataract Refract Surg* Vol. 36, No. 1, (January 2010), pp. 114–120, ISSN: 08863350

Zuclich, J.A. (1989). Ultraviolet-induced photochemical damage in ocular tissues. *Health Phys* Vol. 56, No. 5, (1989), pp. 671–682, ISSN: 00179078